T0245208

The Clinician Educator Guidebook

Laura Weiss Roberts
Editor

The Clinician Educator Guidebook

Steps and Strategies for Advancing Your Career

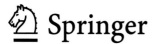 Springer

Editor
Laura Weiss Roberts, MD, MA
Chairman and Katharine Dexter McCormick
  and Stanley McCormick Memorial Professor
Department of Psychiatry and Behavioral Sciences
Stanford University
Stanford, CA, USA

ISBN 978-3-319-27979-4   ISBN 978-3-319-27980-0   (eBook)
DOI 10.1007/978-3-319-27980-0

Library of Congress Control Number: 2016932373

Springer Cham Heidelberg New York Dordrecht London
© Springer International Publishing Switzerland 2016

Printed on acid-free paper

Springer International Publishing AG Switzerland is part of Springer
Science+Business Media (www.springer.com)

For my mother, Anne

Preface

Clinician educators are essential to the social mission of academic medicine: improving the health of the public, serving the needs of communities, and enhancing the well-being of individual patients. Clinician educators provide clinical care and define state-of-the art clinical practice through their efforts in every medical school. Clinician educators are entrusted with teaching, training, and mentoring of students across medicine. Clinician educators also function as team leaders, working with colleagues from across disciplines and professions, and system leaders, helping to transform the quality and broad impact of health care. Clinician educators advance clinical and educational scholarship that, in turn, shapes standards of care and health policy. Much—and much of importance to human health now and in the future—is carried on the shoulders of clinician educator faculty.

Clinician educators are numerous and most are just starting their professional lives in academic medicine. In the most recent count by the Association of American Medical Colleges, the number of clinician educators in US medical schools was nearly double the number of traditional, tenured, or tenure track faculty. Except at the full professor rank, most medical school faculty members are in fact clinician educators. For example, at the assistant professor level in 2014, the number of tenured or tenure track individuals was one-third ($n = 12,734$) the number of faculty *not* on this traditional track ($n = 45,606$) in the USA (https://www.aamc.org/download/420636/data/14table15.pdf). With rare exception, such as at Stanford University where the number of clinician educator faculty surpassed the number of tenure and tenure track faculty in 2013, most medical schools in the USA had more clinician educators than other faculty beginning in the 1990s. Moreover, most medical schools have a "pyramid" structure, with most faculty members being at the instructor and assistant professor ranks. With the current expansion of academic health systems and the growth in the number of medical schools, it is likely that the academic faculty will continue to be largely composed of physicians and other doctoral-level clinicians within their first 10 years after training.

Whether the importance of their mission or the significance of their numbers, clinician-educators have become the foundational academic workforce in the USA and in many countries throughout the world. The critical role of clinician educators and the observation that many of these faculty members are just at the beginning of their careers, taken together, have inspired this book, *The Clinician Educator "Survival" Guide*. Early career clinicians often feel overwhelmed by the newness and breadth of responsibilities that go with their first faculty job. Years of training may have honed their clinical strengths and competencies, but interviewing for a job? Giving a large lecture in front of dozens of students? Using technology to enhance their learners' experience? Reviewing a manuscript for a scientific journal? Putting together an educator's portfolio? Building a national reputation? These aspects of the clinician educator role on a medical school faculty may seem intimidating, particularly as they may not have been addressed at any point in medical school, residency, or fellowship.

The Clinician Educator Guidebook thus provides specific and valuable guidance to foster the success and, I hope, fulfillment of clinician educators in initiating and sustaining their professional lives in academic medicine. This guidebook, which derived from a larger text, *The Academic Medicine Handbook*, centers specifically on the issues of clinician educators.

The guidebook focuses on how to establish the *foundation for an academic career*. Illustrative chapters in this domain include how to interview for a first faculty position, how to prepare a robust curriculum vitae, how to evaluate a letter of offer, and how to understand the process of academic promotion.

The guidebook also highlights the acquisition and refinement of *essential academic skills* for clinician educators relating to education, scholarship, and clinical care. Examples related to educational skills include on how to give a lecture, how to approach clinical supervision, how to incorporate technology in educational innovation, and how to give feedback. In the area of scholarship, the guidebook includes chapters on how to write a case report, how to review a manuscript, and how to build a national reputation for academic promotion. Chapters pertaining to clinical care include how to maintain excellent clinical documentation, how to evaluate clinical research, and how to avoid medicolegal problems.

Perhaps most importantly, this guidebook also gives careful attention to considerations that will help early career clinician educator faculty preserve a sense of *academic purpose and a healthy life balance* as they navigate the demands of their professional and personal lives.

Clinician educators matter to their patients and their students, and their impact is felt throughout every medical school. Clinician educators represent an early career academic workforce; they carry great responsibility for delivering health care, serving as educators, and advancing the field of clinical medicine just as they are getting established in their professional lives. This guidebook is designed as a resource for these dedicated and effortful faculty colleagues who play such an essential role in academic medicine.

Stanford, CA, USA   Laura Weiss Roberts, MD, MA

Acknowledgement

With sincere thanks I wish to acknowledge Katie Ryan, M.A., and Ann Tennier, ELS, for their expertise and assistance in preparing this book.

Contents

Contributors

Richard Balon, M.D. Departments of Psychiatry and Behavioral Neurosciences and Anesthesiology, Wayne State University School of Medicine, Detroit, MI, USA

Liliana Kalogjera Barry, M.D. Department of Psychiatry and Behavioral Medicine, Medical College of Wisconsin, Milwaukee, WI, USA

Amy Becker, M.D. Department of Psychiatry and Behavioral Sciences, Children's Hospital Colorado, Anschutz Medical Campus, Aurora, CO, USA

Eugene Beresin, M.D. Department of Psychiatry, Massachusetts General Hospital, McLean Hospital and Harvard Medical School, Boston, MA, USA

Justin A. Birnbaum, M.D. Department of Psychiatry and Behavioral Sciences, Stanford University, Stanford, CA, USA

Robert Boland, M.D. Division of Biology and Medicine, Department of Psychiatry and Human Behavior, Brown University, Providence, RI, USA

Linda M. Boxer, M.D., Ph.D. Department of Medicine, Stanford University, Stanford, CA, USA

Judith P. Cain Department of Medicine, Stanford University, Stanford, CA, USA

Michael I. Casher, M.D. Department of Psychiatry, University of Michigan Health System, Ann Arbor, MI, USA

Carlyle H. Chan, M.D. Department of Psychiatry and Behavioral Medicine, Medical College of Wisconsin, Milwaukee, WI, USA

Robert Chayer, M.D. Department of Psychiatry and Behavioral Medicine, Medical College of Wisconsin, Milwaukee, WI, USA

Sallie G. DeGolia, M.P.H., M.D. Department of Psychiatry and Behavioral Sciences, Stanford University Hospital and Clinics, Stanford, CA, USA

Laura B. Dunn, M.D. Department of Psychiatry, University of California, San Francisco, San Francisco, CA, USA

Sara R. Figueroa, M.D. Department of Psychiatry, University of Michigan, Ann Arbor, MI, USA

Michelle Goldsmith, M.D., M.A. Division of Child and Adolescent Psychiatry, Department of Psychiatry and Behavioral Health Sciences, Lucile Packard Children's Hospital/Stanford Hospital and Clinics, Stanford, CA, USA

Thomas W. Heinrich, M.D., F.A.P.M. Department of Psychiatry and Behavioral Medicine, Medical College of Wisconsin, Milwaukee, WI, USA

Michael D. Jibson, M.D., Ph.D. Department of Psychiatry, University of Michigan Health System, Ann Arbor, MI, USA

Heather Kenna, M.A. Department of Psychiatry and Behavioral Sciences, Stanford University, Stanford, CA, USA

Jennifer R. Kogan, M.D. Department of Medicine, Perelman School of Medicine at the University of Pennsylvania, Philadelphia, PA, USA

Jon A. Lehrmann, M.D. Department of Psychiatry and Behavioral Medicine, Medical College of Wisconsin, Milwaukee, WI, USA

John Luo, M.D. Department of Psychiatry, UCLA Semel Institute for Neuroscience and Human Behavior, Los Angeles, CA, USA

Christine Moutier, M.D. Department of Psychiatry, University of California, San Diego, School of Medicine, La Jolla, CA, USA

Andrew Norton, M.D. Department of Clinical Medicine, Medical College of Wisconsin, Milwaukee, WI, USA

Laura Weiss Roberts, M.D., M.A. Department of Psychiatry and Behavioral Sciences, Stanford University School of Medicine, Stanford, CA, USA

Deborah Simpson, Ph.D. Academic Administration, Aurora Health Care, Milwaukee, WI, USA

Upinder Singh, M.D. Department of Microbiology and Immunology, Stanford University, Stanford, CA, USA

Department of Medicine, Stanford University, Stanford, CA, USA

David K. Stevenson, M.D. Department of Pediatrics, Stanford University School of Medicine, Stanford, CA, USA

Teddy D. Warner, Ph.D. Department of Family and Community Medicine, University of New Mexico School of Medicine, Albuquerque, NM, USA

Joel Yager, M.D. Department of Psychiatry, University of Colorado School of Medicine, Aurora, CO, USA

Sidney Zisook, M.D. Department of Psychiatry, University of California, San Francisco, CA, USA

Veterans Affairs San Diego Healthcare System and Veterans Medical and Research Foundation, La Jolla, CA, USA

How to Find Your Path in Academic Medicine

Laura Weiss Roberts

> *Although the world is full of suffering, it is full also of the overcominvg of it.*
>
> Helen Keller

Academic medicine exists to create a better future for all of humanity. Medical school faculty fulfill this awesome responsibility through present-day effort in five interdependent realms: advancing science, engaging in clinical innovation and service, fostering multidisciplinary education, collaborating to address societal needs, and nurturing leadership and professionalism. Faculty investigators seek new knowledge to help understand the biological basis of health and disease as well as the psychological, cultural, and social determinants of illness. Academic clinicians apply scientific evidence to help individual patients, to establish better practices, and to create effective systems of care for entire populations. Teachers teach. Medical school educators impart knowledge, build competencies, and inspire students across

L.W. Roberts, M.D., M.A. (✉)
Department of Psychiatry and Behavioral Sciences, Stanford University School of Medicine, 401 Quarry Road, Stanford, CA, USA
e-mail: RobertsL@stanford.edu

© Springer International Publishing Switzerland 2016
L.W. Roberts (ed.), *The Clinician Educator Guidebook*,
DOI 10.1007/978-3-319-27980-0_1

the many disciplines of the health professions. Faculty work with diverse partners to define and take on concerns affecting the health of communities, whether local or global. Medical school faculty, in turn, help cultivate the next generation of leaders— people who will be prepared to offer expertise and wise judgment in broad policy efforts, scientific inquiry, and organizational responses to issues of importance to human health. Through these efforts, individually and collectively, academic faculty members have stepped forward to address vast health problems that do and will affect all people. On the shoulders of academic medicine rides the hope that the world's next generation will live better lives and endure fewer burdens of suffering, disability, and premature mortality.

When entering the profession of academic medicine, it is clear that the path ahead will thus be one of great purpose and hard work. Harder to discern at the outset are three other aspects of a career in academic medicine that are immensely valued by experienced faculty. First, the work itself is creative and complex. Second, the colleagues are extraordinary. And, third, the environment of academic medicine continuously—perhaps relentlessly—causes faculty members to question, to learn, and to extend themselves. *Meaning, effort, creativity, colleagueship*, and *growth*. These elements define the experience of a life dedicated to academic medicine and, taken together, they give rise to careers of unimagined achievement and distinct worth for those who choose this path.

> *A hero is someone who understands the responsibility that comes with his freedom.*
>
>   Bob Dylan

So, how does one choose the path of academic medicine? For some, the aspirational "calling" of helping humanity through discovery or healing will draw them to this field. For many, the love of teaching makes alternative careers—a future without connection to students each day—far less compelling. For others, academic medicine will provide the optimal, most exciting, or only settings for their scientific work. For some "bitten by the bug" of academic medicine, the opportunity to pursue the multiple missions of doing science, caring for patients, teaching, collaborating, and leading plaited as one cohesive endeavor will be irresistible. And for yet others, entering academic medicine may simply feel intuitive and logical—encouraged by their mentors and surrounded by friends, moving from the role as student to faculty member in a familiar context becomes an obvious "next step" in their careers. Perhaps all of these influences have some part in the decisions of students to choose academic medicine.

Whatever the reasons, my sense is that nearly all early-career faculty members experience, as I did, an unsettling combination of feeling overly schooled and, yet, still underprepared. Decades of formal education, as it turns out, are insufficient for some of the unexpected and labor-intensive everyday duties of the instructor/assistant professor, such as writing letters of recommendation, sitting on committees or, worse, seeking committee approvals, formatting one's curriculum vitae, obtaining a "360" evaluation, undergoing compliance audits, fulfilling quality performance metrics, and the like. These tasks are not among those that an early academic thinks of when aspiring to better the human condition. Moreover, the dynamics among the faculty may be rather unexpected. Rather. The esteem, as well as the size of office or laboratory and financial compensation, accorded to an early-career faculty member may also seem just a bit thin after all the years of training. Managing these duties and dynamics and becoming a graceful self-advocate are, one quickly learns, essential to one's success in an academic career. Without some savvy in handling these "fundamentals" in the culture of medical schools, it will be difficult to turn to the bigger work of academic medicine.

Recognition of the importance of these basic, but typically untaught, skills for faculty members across academic medicine serves as the origin of this handbook. The text is organized into eight sections that encompass major domains, duties, and developmental aspects of faculty life. The sections are the following: approaching the profession of academic medicine, getting established, approaching work with colleagues, writing and evaluating manuscripts, conducting empirical research, developing administrative skills, advancing along academic paths, and ensuring personal well-being. Every section will be salient for all academic faculty members—the clinical educator should understand the process that translational scientist colleagues undergo in competing for research grants, for example, and the laboratory scientist should understand the nature of bedside teaching. Such understanding will foster collegiality and it will ensure greater fairness in accomplishing the many citizenship tasks of academic environments, such as when serving on a Promotion and Tenure (or "P & T") committee. The subjects of individual chapters are wide-ranging, derived from my own observations and impressions of what early career faculty "need to know" to navigate the course ahead. Examples of a chapter from each section include how to manage time effectively, how to give a lecture, how to approach the relationship with a mentor, how to write for publication, how to prepare a first grant application, how to negotiate, how to develop a national reputation, and how to manage personal finances. My hope in envisioning and assembling this handbook is that it will assist faculty to be effective and personally fulfilled as they progress through their careers in academic medicine.

Whatever you are, be a good one.

Abraham Lincoln

People who flourish in academic medicine possess certain qualities that allow them to adapt to the diverse and specific ecologies of medical school environments. Years ago Hilty and I observed that our most successful colleagues have several common attributes—beyond having a sense of purpose and the willingness to work hard, they are creative, organized, and tenacious; they foster good will; and they are open to opportunity [1]. As I have seen exceptional careers become damaged, and devastated, in my 19 years as an academic faculty member, I have come to understand that professional integrity, presupposed in the prior list, should be made explicit as a "necessary precondition" for effective academic careers. With experience in leadership roles, I also now include among the characteristics of the strongest faculty the ability to communicate the value of one's work to others and awareness of one's limitations and willingness to compensate, adapt, or reposition accordingly. Knowledge of the overall organization and governance of medical schools and understanding of how medical school realities are shaped by county, state, and federal resources, regulatory agencies, and public policy are also qualities that help faculty do well as they mature within the field. Dedication to the success of others within an academic organization (students, staff, peers, near-peers, or deans) and outside of the academic organization (affiliated institutions, community partners, professional colleagues, or governmental or nongovernmental entities) is another discernible quality of great academic faculty members. All of these characteristics allow a faculty member to thrive in medical school environments, advancing their careers but also supporting the value of these organizations in society.

Indeed, though they represent the "universe" for academic faculty, medical schools are relatively few in number and vary greatly. The Association of American Medical Colleges (AAMC, www.aamc.org) is an organization that represents all of the accredited medical schools in the USA and Canada, their major teaching hospitals and health systems, and key academic and scientific societies in the two countries. At the time of this writing, the AAMC has 137 medical schools in the USA and 17 in Canada, with eight more schools launched and moving toward accreditation by the Liaison Committee on Medical Education, a joint endeavor of the AAMC and the American Medical Association. The AAMC estimates that 128,000 faculty members, 75,000 medical students, and 110,000 resident physicians work within these academic medical organizations. Given that the population of the United States today is estimated to be 313.6 million people and of Canada is 33.5 million people, the number of medical schools is small by any count and the ratio of faculty-to-general population is strikingly low. Keeping the academic workforce robust, given its responsibilities to the many people it serves, is thus essential.

Medical schools must meet clear standards, but are quite different in their scope of activities, priorities, settings, finances, governance, and cultures. All provide high-quality education, though through remarkably diverse curricula. All must have teaching-related clinical services in general and specialty areas. Some medical schools have robust federal research funding for science, whereas others have nearly none. Some medical schools are financially sturdy while others find themselves frequently near fiscal collapse, trading program closure for the opportunity for the organization to survive another week. Some medical schools have as their primary task educating rural care providers to serve the health of neighboring communities, and some see their foremost duty as driving forward the most innovative basic and translational science that will transform all of our current understanding of human health and disease. Some medical schools ("medical colleges") are independent and free-standing, and others reside on a university campus embedded in a health sciences center with companion nursing, dental, and other health professional schools. Culturally, some medical schools take great pride in their elite standing while others, some of the best schools among them, have a much more down-to-earth nature.

Such diverse environments suggest the value of a diverse set of people suited to the work of academic medicine. Scientists, clinicians, teachers, leaders, and "mosaics" all belong. Success as a faculty member will thus involve looking for the "best fit" between the person and the organization and, more specifically, the person at a particular point in his or her professional development and the organization at a particular point in its history. Extraordinary ("top tier") institutions can help advance stellar careers through exceptional mentors and facilities, but for some early-career faculty it may be difficult to get the recognition and opportunities that they would receive as a "bigger fish" in a "smaller pond." More modest institutions may not have the resources to afford the larger commitments needed by their talented, let alone their "superstar," faculty, however. Institutional history is also relevant in that academic entities that have grown through investments in basic science or, alternatively, in clinical expansion are likely to adhere to their past successes in future decisions. Academic programs that have thrived by taking "high-risk, high-gain" commitments are likely to be bolder whereas fiscally strapped entities or those that have, let's say, just undergone investigation by the federal government for human subjects compliance concerns may be very conservative in their decision-making. These factors, though they seem far-removed from the everyday life of the individual faculty member, shape the milieu and can greatly influence the academic work that each person undertakes.

In thinking through whether a particular academic setting will help support the development of one's academic life, an early career faculty member should look for several features of the environment. The most basic elements include the presence of a mentor or mentors to help guide and some basic resources necessary to complete the academic work of the faculty member, e.g., access to a laboratory, access to a methodologist or quantitative expert, access to patient populations, access to students, and the like. Collaborative colleagues will enrich the academic environment further. If the productivity and workload expectations are rigorous but reasonable, and if there is a supervisor or even an opinion leader who values one's work, then the environment may well be sufficient. If there is a special aspect of an environment that is more important than all of the rest, in my view, it is whether there is a positive culture of curiosity, exploration, opportunity, and forgiveness that allows faculty members to learn, to expand their expertise, and to take on new responsibilities. One caveat: if the constellation of duties undertaken by the faculty member is not well-thought through, even the optimal academic environment will not support academic success. Carefully evaluating what is possible in the pairing of a faculty member and the institution/institutional role is therefore essential.

Beyond thinking about the context of one academic program or one organization, it is also valuable to entertain the possibility of making certain key moves over the course of one's professional life. These moves may occur within an institution, for instance, in seeking a new leadership role, or involve transitioning to a new faculty post at a new institution. Both kinds of change can be disruptive, and no one recommends "job-hopping." That said, intentional and well-judged moves both can bring immense opportunities for faculty members as well as the institutional environments in which they serve.

Far and away the best prize that life has to offer is the chance to work hard at work worth doing.

Theodore Roosevelt

The profession of academic medicine requires constant sustenance and renewal. For academic faculty, it is a time in history that holds the greatest promise in terms of scientific discovery, clinical innovation, educational advances, mutualism with other societal stakeholders, and true leadership. Each individual entering academic medicine can anticipate an exceptional career—one that is rich and exciting professionally and fulfilling personally. Our profession is nevertheless fragile. Resource concerns, erosion of the public trust, and inadequate numbers of people entering and remaining in scientific and clinical careers, in particular, threaten academic medicine. The significance of the fragility does not pertain to the interests of individual institutions or what may be perceived as petty concerns of "guild" subspecialties or disciplines—the real meaning is far greater because the consequences reach forward to the future. Our capacity to better the lives of people throughout the world, and shape the health of their children, will be lessened if academic medicine is allowed to languish. More positively stated, though it has been in existence for less than a century, the modern model of academic medicine has already brought about enduring good for humankind and, though the specific configuration of organizations may evolve, its value is certain to continue.

Inspiring exceptional young physicians and scientists, supporting them as they find their professional "calling," and fostering their development in academic medicine, taken together, therefore represent sincere commitments for our field. I said at the beginning of this chapter that academic medicine exists to help humanity, but it exists too because of the people who have committed their lives to it. For this reason, I end this initial chapter of *The Academic Medicine Handbook: A Guide to Achievement and Fulfillment for Academic Faculty* with a statement of appreciation for our early career colleagues, individuals who have already sacrificed and accomplished much and are choosing to join the authors of this volume on a professional path in academic medicine. We welcome you to this endeavor, the work of imagining and creating a better future—and we thank you for stepping forward.

Words to the Wise
- Consider the five missions of academic medicine—where do your interests, strengths, and commitments fit?
- Take a good look at your colleagues and mentors: What can you learn from their career choices? What can you learn from their successes and failures?
- What practical skills do you need to progress in your career?
- How does your department compare with other departments nationally?
- What future do you envision in academic medicine?

Ask Your Mentor or Colleagues
- What kind of academic setting might be best for me?
- How can I prepare myself for the everyday duties of a new career in academic medicine?
- What are my strengths? Do I have limitations that I should try to remedy or compensate for?
- What are the predictable choice-points in an academic career path?
- Who else should I be talking with to help me think about my career and professional growth?

Reference

1. Roberts LW, Hilty DM. Approaching your academic career. In: Roberts LW, Hilty DM, editors. Handbook of career development in academic psychiatry and behavioral sciences. Arlington, VA: American Psychiatric Press, Inc; 2006. p. 3–10.

How to Build the Foundation for a Successful Career in Academia

2

Upinder Singh and Linda M. Boxer

It is the ultimate goal for many who go to medical or graduate school—joining the faculty ranks of an academic institution. For many, this seems an uphill battle, and financial, social, and lifestyle pressures are causing increasing number of graduates to abandon this goal. However, such a goal remains attainable, worthwhile, and desirable and offers a challenging career filled with great rewards. A career in academic medicine is never routine or boring and provides enormous flexibility, yet enough intellectual stimulation and opportunities for growth to sustain interest and excitement for a lifetime.

In this chapter we outline some strategies that can pave the path to success while keeping in mind that each academic physician will have a unique and personal journey. Some factors that predict success are so obvious as to seem formulaic and repetitive, but still deserve discussion. Absolute requirements for the job are (1) possessing motivation and willingness to work hard, (2) being focused on goals in an efficient and organized manner that allows one to set priorities and achieve measurable success in them, (3) being prepared to network in one's field and obtain funding, and (4) having adequate protected time and aligning with the goals of the department and

L.M. Boxer, M.D., Ph.D. (✉)
Department of Medicine, Stanford University, 269 Campus Drive,
Stanford, CA, USA
e-mail: lboxer@stanford.edu

© Springer International Publishing Switzerland 2016
L.W. Roberts (ed.), *The Clinician Educator Guidebook*,
DOI 10.1007/978-3-319-27980-0_2

institution. Other skills are more nuanced and not so immediately obvious and relate to the ability to get the first academic job and to grow and mature in the position. These skills include the ability to deal with challenges and take risks and to understand one's strengths and weaknesses and learn from mistakes. Additionally, the ability to find mentors for different aspects of one's career and to be flexible enough to accommodate new opportunities and challenges is key to continued professional development and satisfaction.

Is This the Right Faculty Position?

In searching for a faculty position, a key predictor of future success is alignment of one's goals with those of the department and institution. Determine what an institution values and whether those priorities fit your short- and long-term goals. If your interests are not in line with the institutional vision, do not take a position just because you are enamored by the aura of the institution. Before accepting a faculty position, it is critical to agree with your chief or chair on how your effort will be divided among the three major academic missions of research, clinical care, and teaching. You will most likely spend significantly more time in one of the three missions. Likewise, the faculty position will be structured with a major focus on one of the missions. To accept a position that is not designed to allow you to spend the preponderance of your time on the mission that is of most importance to you and your career development is a recipe for disappointment and failure. In your discussions on the faculty position, be clear about the expectations that the chief or the chair has for what constitutes success. Spend the time to develop a realistic budget for your research needs for at least the first 3 years, and negotiate with the chief or the chair for this support. You will also need salary support during this time. Ask to see the offer in writing and make certain it is clear. Do not be afraid to ask for the resources and protected time that you need.

Once at the right place, finding colleagues who have similar aspirations will provide the essential intellectual support needed to develop your own scholarship. We do not live in a vacuum and certainly cannot succeed in one. Getting adequate support to develop your scholarship (protected time and resources being two important considerations) are key factors, as are clear expectations of how your time as a new faculty member will be spent (e.g., what proportion will be research, clinical, teaching, administrative). Many early-career faculty fall into the trap of overcommitting to too many service tasks early in their careers. The desire to be a good citizen is laudable, but the necessity to protect one's time during the early years of establishing a research program cannot be overstated.

Establishing Your Identity

Your research mentor has been a great guide for you and helped you develop as a scientist, writer, thinker, manager, and maybe even leader. However, as in all relationships, there is a time when some important and tough conversations must occur.

> Your angle: I am going out into the world and need to establish my scientific identity and I want to talk about how I will separate from you—what scientific projects would be yours and what work will be mine?
>
> Your mentor's angle: Great! I am excited for you to begin your own career. But your work has been some of the best in my lab—I am not sure how much of it I can give to you!

In the ideal world, the mentor's and trainee's goals, visions, and plans are completely aligned, but in the real world, where science is tough, funding difficult, and the competitive spirit drives all of us, the issue of separation and differentiation can often be challenging. To avoid misunderstandings, the best approach is to (1) have frank and honest conversations, (2) broach the topic early, (3) set up expectations on both sides, and (4) have regular follow-up. Another consideration is to have a specific time period when you are still working closely with a mentor but you are pursuing an independent project. This can be best accomplished when you have independent funding and will depend on the collaborative and collegial nature of your mentor. Keep in mind that science is difficult to predict. Even if your mentor and you agree to divide work, eventually your mentor's projects may collide with yours. Be prepared for this situation, but do not let fear of it hold you back from tackling the best and most interesting scientific questions. If your mentor has taught you well, you are prepared with the skills to be a friendly colleague, collaborator, and even competitor!

One special consideration is when you take a faculty position at the same institution as your mentor. Although such an arrangement has many advantages (e.g., you are already familiar with the environment, have scientific colleagues around you whom you know, can easily set up your own lab, and it is easier on you and your family not to move across the country), one disadvantage is continued association with your former mentor. In the eyes of your colleagues, will you be a new faculty colleague or simply the great senior postdoc of your mentor? This perception is not absolute and can be overcome, but you will have to make and follow a plan to overcome this perception successfully. Keep in mind that this separation is not just for the sake of your ego—it is for the sake of your career. When the time arrives for decisions on promotion and tenure, you will be judged on how you differentiated from your former mentor and whether you have established a research program that is unique, independent, and additive to the program of your mentor. In other words, what do you bring to the table that your mentor did not?

Setting Priorities and Focusing on Them

Once you have navigated the first few busy (and stressful!) years of life as a new faculty member, your thoughts will soon turn to the next steps—reappointment, promotion, and tenure. Have a discussion with your chief or chair on the criteria for reappointment and promotion. Different faculty lines are designed to emphasize each of the three academic missions, and the requirements for promotion will differ among the lines. You have previously made certain to enter the line that is the best fit for your goals and interests. Therefore, the criteria for promotion will likely align with your priorities. Once you have an understanding of the criteria for promotion, ask your mentors for their advice and feedback on what your priorities should be. Know the metrics on which you will be judged so that you can determine your readiness for and success in being promoted. Get as many perspectives as possible—ask, ask, ask. Ask those around you who have recently navigated this hurdle, ask mentors and supervisors what areas you should prioritize, and ask scientific colleagues for their insight and guidance. Among the abundance of advice you receive, common themes will emerge—keep those in mind as you set your goals and priorities.

It is very important to have protected time during your first several years on the faculty. Protected time will allow you to develop your scholarship, clinical practice, and/or teaching. When you are asked to take on a new project or assignment, consider how this work will help you attain your goals. Although some good citizenship activities are desirable and necessary, it is not reasonable to expect an early-career faculty member to engage heavily in these types of activities. With the advice and support of your mentors, determine which activities will be most beneficial for your career development without taking too much time away from your academic mission endeavors. Be focused and merciless about committing to new assignments or projects. Will they help or hinder you in your long-term goals? Taking on new projects that will ultimately help you is not being selfish—it is being smart.

Mentors, Mentors, and More Mentors

The importance of mentors as key predictors of success cannot be overstated. Academic medicine is complex, and listening to the advice of others who know how to negotiate the course will help ensure your success. You cannot have too many mentors, but do not expect them to seek you out. Go and find them. Keep in mind that you will need mentors for many aspects of your academic life— three areas that are the most obvious are research, clinical, and teaching. However, academic physicians also need and benefit from mentors in other areas—maintaining work–life balance, writing well and effectively, public speaking, and so on. It is valuable to have a mentoring team—one mentor does not have to fill all these varied roles. Keep in mind that your need for mentoring will also change over time, and the input and guidance you needed as a new faculty member will be vastly different from the guidance you need as you take on leadership roles. A good place to start in the search for mentors is with your chief or chair and/or your assigned mentor. Several of your mentors will likely be at your institution, but do not limit your mentorship support to colleagues at the same institution. For example, you may need to identify a mentor for your research from investigators in the same research area as yours, and it is quite possible that there will be no one at your home institution in your research field. Your research mentor from your time as a trainee may be able to assist with finding a mentor at another institution. Many institutions offer formal training in teaching skills, which is a valuable resource. It may be possible to identify a mentor to assist with developing your teaching abilities from among the faculty who participate in the training program. As you engage in clinical care, you will likely identify more senior clinical faculty who can serve as mentors and role models.

The best mentors provide honest feedback and advice, pointing to areas for improvement as well as helping you navigate the maze of academic medicine. A mentor who can identify areas for improvement and provide support and advice during the process is very skilled, and you will be fortunate to have such mentors. Stay flexible and be open-minded—many informal mentoring relationships can develop with senior colleagues. Although one does not often consider the need for support and advice on how to become a mentor as one begins a career in academic medicine, mentorship is an important requirement that will develop as you start to work with trainees in research and/or clinical care. One often unrecognized but great benefit to having wonderful mentors is that they can help you develop your mentoring skills. What aspects of a mentor were fantastic; what other habits were less than ideal? Look back at your experience and learn from it. Take the best of what you experienced and contribute to the next generation by being a great mentor. Many faculty members find the process of mentoring and developing early-career colleagues to be one of the most rewarding aspects of a career in academic medicine.

"Tooting Your Own Horn": Be Your Own Best Advocate

As scientists we are often taught to be modest—for example, analyze the data carefully, do not overcall your results, and do not be too broad and generalize beyond what this experiment shows. Although that approach works well in science, it can also hinder you when it is time for you to "sell" yourself. Remember that although your mentor, chief or chair, and other colleagues may do their best to promote you, the person who can best "pitch your product" is you. You need to be your own best advocate. Your job is to do great science, be a good mentor, communicate your data effectively and energetically, and network well with colleagues and collaborators. In addition, you need to keep track of what you have done for the institution (e.g., invited seminars, teaching responsibilities, committees, clinical work, mentoring students) and have that data for your supervisor. Having a systematic way to keep track of what you have contributed to the academic mission of your institution is key. You must toot your own horn—or at least provide the data to your chair so that he or she can toot a horn on your behalf!

I Do Not Look Like Other Faculty Members

The special challenges of being a faculty member as an underrepresented minority or a woman deserve mention. Identifying people whom we look like or to whom we aspire to emulate are important factors in shaping our thoughts about our potential. Seeing women faculty who have successful academic careers, handle work–life balance, and succeed in leadership positions gives the younger generation of women confidence that they too can have this career and be successful at it. For an underrepresented minority faculty member, the importance of finding others who look like him or her or have similar cultural backgrounds is also essential. As with many situations, success breeds success. An institution that has shown the commitment to recruit and retain underrepresented minority and women faculty members will have greater success with recruiting new faculty members in these categories. The awareness of the importance of having a rich, blended faculty at all ranks has been steadily increasing, and most nationally ranked institutions have special programs focused on the recruitment and retention of faculty who are women and underrepresented minorities.

What About My Significant Other?

It is now the norm that recruitment of a faculty member will involve assistance with career opportunities for his or her significant other. It may be a dual recruitment into the same department or different departments at the academic institution or help with locating an appropriate position in the area. This recruitment issue is particularly challenging not only for the couple but also for the institution. Many academic institutions have a person or an office to assist with issues related to dual-career couples. A significant question for the faculty applicant is when to raise this topic. As a candidate for a position, you should not be asked whether you have a significant other or family. You need to determine the appropriate time to begin this discussion. It may be reasonable to discuss this topic with the chair or the chief at the second visit or at the time you receive a formal offer. You and your significant other should decide in advance what assistance is needed, what kinds of positions would be appropriate for the other member of the couple, and what compromises you are each willing to accept. Dual-career couples face challenges at every stage of their training and career as they move forward in their professional lives. They may undergo a number of moves to different institutions, and these moves are often driven by the career of one member of the couple. How to balance the effect of a move on the career of the other member of the couple is difficult and must be handled with sensitivity on the part of all involved. This is another area in which mentors can be very helpful, especially those mentors who are members of dual-career couples themselves.

When Mistakes Happen

As accomplished as you are for winning the search for the faculty position, you will have areas of weakness or limitations that can be worked on and improved, just as everyone has. It is helpful to ask your mentors and others who know you well in different settings to assist you in evaluating your strengths and areas that require improvement. As you begin to work on your weaknesses, do not neglect your strengths. These are the personal characteristics that got you to where you are now and serve as the foundation of your success—do not neglect them, but enhance them and add to them. These can continue to be built upon, and you want to maintain them as areas that are strong for you. Once you have identified some limitations or weaknesses, work with your mentors on strategies to deal with them or to turn them into strengths. As an example, stubbornness is usually identified as a trait that is limiting, but you can learn to develop this trait into persistence, which is much more useful and can be a positive force.

As an early-career faculty member, you will feel the need to appear confident and knowledgeable. We all hope that each step along the path of an academic career will be filled with successes, but you will undoubtedly make mistakes along the way. You may identify a mistake or someone else may point it out to you. In either case, the best approach is to admit the mistake and work with your mentors to determine what you can learn from it. With this knowledge you can move forward and avoid making a similar mistake. The most worrisome aspect of mistakes is to fail to learn from them and to continue to err in the same way. Understanding your strengths and weaknesses and learning from your mistakes are crucial to continued personal and professional growth. To paraphrase a famous quote: those who cannot learn from failure are condemned to repeat it.

Continue to Take Risks

What brought you to where you are now was the ability to take scientific risks, think in new ways, and ask the big and important scientific questions. Creativity is valued in academic medicine, and success often results from the use of novel approaches. Once you are in a faculty role, it is important not to lose this perspective. Although the initial focus may be in pursuing some safer route, one needs to be creative, willing to try new approaches, and open to new experiences. Having a mixture of high-risk/high-reward projects in addition to those that are likely to succeed is generally the best approach. The safer projects are those that are guaranteed to get papers published and lay the foundation for grants and funding. Advice from an experienced research mentor will be valuable in assessing the balance of research projects in your portfolio. The colleagues that surround us are often catalysts for initiating new projects, and although having plans for your research program is important, it is also important to be ready to take on new opportunities when they present themselves. As we take on each new challenge, we learn from it, grow, improve, and develop.

With your mentors, you will chart a path for success as a new faculty member. Throughout your career, however, you will be presented with opportunities that you did not foresee or necessarily seek. Although these may not be part of your plans for career development, it is essential to remain open to new possibilities. You can assess a new opportunity with the assistance of your mentors and determine whether it is one you choose to pursue. It is important to appraise whether you will thrive in the new role or option, and how it will affect the other areas of your work, including research, clinical care, and teaching. It is beneficial to take on challenges and to learn from them. Clearly, the most important goal of an early-career faculty member is to focus on the three major missions and make the strongest case possible for promotion. Therefore, any new opportunity must be judged in this context.

Work–Life Balance: Do Not Ignore It!

The importance of work–life balance and making time to "recharge" cannot be overstated. Remember, this is a marathon, not a sprint. Everyone needs to have time to recharge, both intellectually and emotionally. People are most creative when they have the mental freedom to think, explore, and ponder. Stifling the creative spirit by not allowing oneself to recharge is a common mistake among young scientists. There cannot be perfect work–life balance in every day, every week, or even every month—months with a grant deadline, for example. A careful self-assessment should be performed on a routine basis so that the balance of work and life is maintained. See what others are doing to maintain some level of harmony and find examples you want—or do not want—to emulate. Then figure out your personal solution. A career in academic medicine, particularly as a new faculty member, comes with substantial pressures and stress. You will need to develop methods to handle stress and maintain a healthy lifestyle. Not all approaches to stress management are healthy. You can learn from your mentors and colleagues how they minimize stress and maintain a healthy balance between work and other aspects of their life. A career in academic medicine can be very rewarding. You have intellectual freedom and can make a positive impact in a number of areas. As a new faculty member, your entire career lies ahead of you. With hard work and support and advice from senior colleagues, you are off to a great start.

Conclusion

It takes an enormous amount of motivation, hard work, perseverance, and determination to reach the point where one is offered a faculty position. However, the hard work is not done, and the next steps (e.g., getting your scholarly program established and productive) are often just as challenging. Apply the same strategies and approaches that got you this far: be efficient; commit to the time it will take to build your career; make plans, including a timeline for obtaining research grants and writing papers; and network with others in your field by going to meetings and interacting with the leaders in your area of scholarship. Your mentors will provide support and advice, but you must be committed to building your career and spending the time that is required for this. When you are at work, maintain your focus on the tasks at hand. Learn to be as efficient as possible, seeking guidance and training with efficiency if necessary. Determine what is important for your career success. Make a timeline for the submission of grants supported by strong preliminary data and for the preparation of manuscripts. Be certain to attend important meetings in your field of scholarship, and make an effort to meet the leaders in the field. Your research mentor can help facilitate these meetings and your invitations to meetings to present your research. Promotion requires visibility in your area of scholarship, and investigators in the field will be asked to critique your scholarship and assess your likelihood for continued success. Maintain time for yourself and your family—and keep your creative spirits flowing. Most important, take time to reflect on why you love the job of academic medicine and enjoy the process!

Words to the Wise
- You cannot have too many mentors.
- Be certain to obtain sufficient protected time to develop scholarship.
- Set priorities and focus on them.
- Make certain your goals fit with those of the department and the institution.
- Success requires motivation and hard work.
- Understand your strengths and weakness and learn from your mistakes.
- Do not be afraid to take risks.
- Do not neglect other aspects of your life; work–life balance is the key to long-term success.

Ask Your Mentor or Colleagues
- Give me honest feedback—how do you think I am doing?
- What are the next steps for my career development?
- What was the biggest mistake you made in your first position?
- What was your best decision in your first position?
- What is the best advice you can give me at this point in my career?
- How do you maintain a balance between work and the rest of your life and how do you deal with stress?

How to Have a Healthy Life Balance as an Academic Physician

3

Christine Moutier

The well-being of physicians has personal, professional, and public health ramifications. A physician's personal health and well-being are not only vital to the individual physician and his or her family members and community but may also affect that physician's life professionally. Moreover, on a larger societal scale, physician wellness also likely serves a critical role in the delivery of high-quality healthcare. When physicians are unwell, the performance of healthcare systems can be negatively affected [1]. Good health and mental well-being contribute to the solid foundation on which physicians can be resilient in the face of challenge and optimally address the many stresses of professional life and clinical work. But even for those physicians who understand this connection and are motivated to improve their situation, the real rub comes in practical obstacles of time and energy. Limitations of time and energy are very real, and after the essential tasks of one's work and personal responsibilities are fulfilled, physicians may feel there is little time left to create change that could lead to improvement in health or well-being. This chapter will provide strategies to address this particularly vexing problem many academic physicians face: how to optimally balance work and personal life to enhance the outcome on both sides.

C. Moutier, M.D. (✉)
Department of Psychiatry, University of California, San Diego, School of Medicine, 9500 Gilman Drive, La Jolla, CA, USA
e-mail: cmoutier@ucsd.edu

© Springer International Publishing Switzerland 2016
L.W. Roberts (ed.), *The Clinician Educator Guidebook*,
DOI 10.1007/978-3-319-27980-0_3

Physician Distress

The literature on physician and trainee distress has shown an association between various forms of distress and both professional commitment and clinical performance. The predicted shortfall of physicians in the workforce is compounded by continued concerns about job satisfaction and intention to leave the profession [2]. Burnout, depressive symptoms, and low quality of life are all too common among resident physicians and have been associated with negative effects on patient care including major medical and medication errors, suboptimal care practices, and decreased patient satisfaction with medical care [3]. Among medical students, burnout has been associated with lower levels of empathy and increased incidence of unprofessional behaviors such as cheating [4]. When burnout is severe and chronic (>12 months) even more severe forms of distress, such as suicidal ideation, occur at higher rates [5]. Unfortunately, physicians have higher rates of completed suicide than their age-matched nonphysician peers [6]. While suicide comprises a narrow and very extreme sequelae of underrecognized, untreated, or undertreated psychiatric illness, it is an important and tragic outcome along the continuum of physician distress.

Efforts in Medical Education

Undergraduate medical education promotes the concept of self-care as a physician's professional responsibility, teaches wellness strategies, attempts to destigmatize mental healthcare, and encourages help-seeking at appropriate times. In 2002 the accrediting body for U.S. medical schools, the Liaison Committee on Medical Education, mandated that medical schools prioritize student wellness by providing education related to well-being and stress management and regular opportunities to participate in activities that promote resilience and optimal physical and mental health. Graduate medical education similarly has made significant changes in the area of resident well-being, originally driven by the need to protect patient safety, but more recently with an integrated concern for both resident well-being and its interconnection with patient care. These efforts have specifically addressed resident sleep and fatigue with changes in the Accreditation Council for Graduate Medical Education regulations in 2003 and 2011 not only limiting work hours but also requiring the monitoring of resident well-being. Medical education and training may be a time when young physicians learn early habits (for good or for bad) and may be particularly sensitive to the informal curriculum of the profession, which has not always promoted the prioritizing of one's own well-being.

Conceptual Framework for Wellness

For a given individual, how does an everyday mishap (e.g., spilt milk) lead to a calm, even compassionate response on 1 day but provoke an irritable outburst on another? Imagine that the myriad of internal human factors (physiologic, psychological, spiritual) that culminate in the most mature intellectual, emotional, and behavioral response in the face of stress can be condensed into one substance, a fuel source if you will, which, if used fully by the mind and heart, lead to the most healthy, optimal, and likely ethical responses to the plethora of stressors that come up in every day personal and professional life of physicians. In a dynamic way, the day-to-day and even moment-to-moment thoughts, ideas, and responses to stress may be viewed in a model akin to a complex mechanical system. This system relies on an adequate fuel source to perform its functions in a streamlined way. In a similar way, an individual's responses are affected by the amount and quality of "reserve fuel" from which to draw. The human coping reservoir depends on positive input (inflow of fuel), negative input (outflow or loss of fuel), and the structure and characteristics of the reservoir itself [7] (see Fig. 3.1).

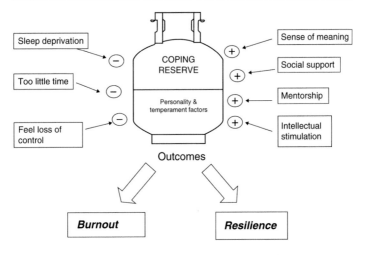

Fig. 3.1 Conceptual model of a coping reservoir. Adapted from [7]

Key Concepts
- *Flourishing*: Optimal state of human existence and functioning, cultivated over a period of time, that encompasses a sense of goodness, generativity, growth, and resilience. An area of study in the field of positive psychology.
- *Burnout*: A response to chronic occupational stress. Tends to occur when workload is high and sense of autonomy, control, and meaning in one's work is low. Consists of a triad of experiences: (1) emotional depletion, (2) sense of detachment, and (3) low sense of achievement.

Internal Structure and Characteristics of the Coping Reservoir

Academic physicians come to the profession of medicine with unique personal characteristics and therefore different strengths and weaknesses. Some are more intrinsically resilient than others and some are more prone to anxiety and depression. This intrinsic "sturdiness" versus "leakiness" of the reservoir is based on a variety of factors including genetics, early childhood, and current environmental factors, and temperament, such as optimism and neuroticism. Physicians tend to be highly driven, conscientious to obsessive, and relatively stoic. While these traits can be positive qualities in a physician, they can also lead to personal suffering.

Depleting Factors (Negative Inputs)

The following areas are common sources of depletion of the coping reservoir, but naturally there are as many unique drains on well-being and resilience as there are individuals.

1. *Stress*: The topic of stress encompasses a vast area and is an unavoidable reality of life for all. Early in medical training, curricular and academic rigors of medical school and residency are easily identified stressors; however, neither education nor stress ends with formal training. Physicians in practice must keep abreast of an ever-enlarging body of skills and knowledge while performing all of the tasks and responsibilities of a busy clinical practice. The struggle for some physicians to keep up-to-date may be squashed by the overwhelming demands of practice. This may be especially true for high-volume, solo, clinical practice environments. This struggle can lead to fears about one's competence on the one hand, or rationalization or even denial of one's deficiencies on the other. There are also common personal psychosocial events which physicians may experience at any age or stage of career. These include personal or family illness, divorce or the break-up of a relationship, death of a loved one, and/or financial problems. The convergence of personal crisis with the steady level of professional stress may lead to a decrement in overall well-being, and in this relatively decompensated state, coping strategies may then deteriorate into less adaptive ones. Maladaptive attempts to cope like using alcohol or drugs (prescription or illicit) obviously pose further risk, such as loss of judgment and legal and/or clinical ramifications. Another pathway that can challenge homeostatic well-being is the occurrence of professional crisis such as a particularly difficult

malpractice suit, interpersonal problems in the workplace, or the jarring experience of having one's clinical competence called into question by a hospital's peer review process or by a licensing board. All of these potential sources of increased stress in the life of a physician can drain the coping reservoir and lead to further distress and/or maladaptive coping.

2. *Anxiety or Internal Conflict*: The experience of doubt or conflicting emotions about aspects of life and one's own decisions is commonplace, germane to a normal neurotic personality structure, and essential to a self-reflective process—important in the practice of medicine. However, if doubt and worry grow into excessive, pathological anxiety, the effect of the anxiety itself can be an extreme drain on fuel/energyconscience or ethical guidelines. (Ironically, excessive worrying is rarely recognized as such by the worrier, perhaps due to the tendency to focus on the perceived problem.) Some physicians may question their choice of specialty or commitment to medicine. If distress deepens, a snowballing process may occur whereby symptoms of anxiety and depression can lead the individual to conclude that medicine or one's choice of specialty were wrong decisions. Reasoning based on negative emotions can result in distorted perceptions and a downward spiral leading to poor performance and worsening depression. Another source of internal conflict comes in the form of the keeping of a personal secret, such as a physician who has made a major medical error, but not acted in accordance with his or her conscience or ethical guidelines, or a gay medical student who has not come out yet to family or community. These secrets tend to weigh heavily as invisible sources of stress, which, when processed and worked through with a mentor or therapist, can lead to the release of an enormous emotional burden.

3. *Demands on time and energy*: There is probably not a single academic physician who has not experienced the challenge of juggling many responsibilities in a finite amount of time: professional responsibilities (clinical, administrative, and/or academic), family, partner, household, friends, and self (e.g., exercise, relaxation/recreation, spiritual practice). Over time, these demands, coupled with fatigue and guilt over unmet obligations can result in burnout, which is characterized by three

criteria: emotional exhaustion ("just going through the motions"); a diminished sense of achievement; and depersonalization (sense of detachment). While time is certainly a finite commodity, and energy may seem to fall into the same category, the energy that fuels resilience can be proactively monitored and replenished. Physicians can learn how to prevent the phenomenon of "running on empty" by understanding the signs of depletion, ideally learning to see it coming in advance and modifying accordingly, and knowing which activities provide the highest level of replenishment. In this way and counter to the prevailing societal view that "life happens to you," individuals can actually exert a reasonable level of control over the outcome of one's own well-being.

Replenishing Factors (Positive Inputs)

Some activities are essential to the basic human needs for rest and replenishment: sleep, good nutrition, and exercise. Perhaps surprisingly though, physicians and students who have high levels of clinical and scientific knowledge to apply to patient care and other professional activities, often need reminders that their own health will be negatively impacted if they shortchange sleep, healthy food, or exercise for long. Other potentially high-impact replenishing factors are included below.

1. *Psychosocial support*: Support can come from many sources within and outside the profession: spouse/partner, family, friends, peers/colleagues, and spiritual support. Psychosocial support can be more formal and provided by counselors, psychotherapists, or executive coaches. Specific groups, such as regional or local professional associations, can provide important support and practical information about how to balance the multiple demands of professional life.
2. *Mentoring*: Mentoring should not stop with the completion of medical training. Of the many important roles mentors fulfill, among the most vital are role modeling and supporting the art of balancing many roles, and recognizing the need for rest and replenishing one's own reservoir. The ideal situation at any given time is to have a mentor or more likely, mentors, who can

advise and consult on a regular or as needed basis, and also to be a mentor to more junior colleagues or trainees.

3. *Experiencing meaning and purpose*: Hard work and fatigue are far more satisfying and positive when they come as a result of investing oneself in something the practitioner finds meaningful and interesting. One challenge is to figure out which activities bring the greatest sense of meaning and purpose. For some physicians, a moment of connection or the act of helping a patient or student are extremely meaningful; for others, building or improving a healthcare system brings a greater sense of purpose. Self-awareness of which activities provide the greatest sense of wholeness, in professional or personal life, does not necessarily come automatically or completely intuitively but, rather, benefits from introspection and an attempt to objectively be a student of oneself and one's own life. How has it worked in the past? The experiences that had the highest emotional impact or clarified a particular career direction are probably still the types of activities that would serve as fuel for optimal coping in the present day. For many in academic medicine, the "meaning" of medicine is amplified through work as a clinician or teacher. Additionally, the arts and humanities significantly enhance life, and more specifically, advancing knowledge in the history of medicine or bioethics can be especially rewarding.

The Nature of the Coping Reservoir

The coping reservoir, like all human systems, is dynamic: ebbing and flowing, rising and falling over time. The goal is to keep the reservoir replenished. Given the burdens placed upon physicians and the inherent variability of individuals' resilience, it is probably unreasonable to expect the reservoir to be continuously full, brimming with high-octane fuel. Still, we must strive to keep the reservoir full *enough*.

Failure to keep the coping reservoir full enough can lead to cynicism, pessimism, frustration, burnout, and, eventually, depression. While the topic of suicide prevention in physicians warrants much greater focus, the prevention of depression and recognition and treatment of symptoms of depression are known to be the best ways to prevent suicide. By finding ways to most effectively replenish the coping reservoir, resilience can flourish and, to the degree that is possible, suffering and disability can be prevented.

How to Keep the Reservoir Full (Enough)

Might it be possible to increase well-being, to diminish dysphoria, to feel more whole and present in the moment? And in a dynamic way over time, is it possible to adjust the positive and negative inputs to prevent burnout or crisis and optimize overall flourishing? If so, without necessarily changing the external circumstances of one's life, can an individual impact these outcomes? It *is* possible, even in the life of a physician, which tends to be tilted heavily in the direction of professional time and energy demands.

A proactive approach to keeping one's coping reservoir full is optimal if not required. Left unattended, most will find that as a matter of time and life's natural demands, the reservoir will drain, and the experience of running on empty leads to real consequences. Proactive approaches include the following:

1. Use a calendar as a tool to proactively plan healthy activities. While simple, scheduling health-promoting "nonnegotiables," e.g., sleep, exercise, quality time for important relationships, other high-impact activity outside of medicine, may allow professional demands and scheduling to be more balanced.
2. Have an inner circle of 1–3 trusted individuals with whom you can safely disclose concerns, e.g., partner, friend, mentor, colleague, therapist, pastor.
3. Establish care with a physician if you don't have one.
4. Pay attention to red flags: irritability and losing one's temper are often the first signs of imbalance; short-term memory slips are another sign of increased stress. Big red flags include increasing alcohol consumption or self-prescribing.
5. Take at least one real vacation each year.
6. Develop a list of priorities. This can be used to shape your decisions about how to approach which activities/relationships can be diminished versus increased. After creating your list, you may realize that a particular activity is actually lower on the list than it used to be, e.g., research or a relationship, and the

acknowledgement of that change or revelation of an erroneous assumption may be instructive, allowing you to spend less time doing, or even take out, an activity.

7. Embrace the truth that you don't have to do and be everything at all times. In other words, career and life have natural phases, and with each changing phase, you can decide which set of roles is most important, appropriate, and feasible.

8. Be as compassionate with yourself as you would be with a loved one. This includes forgiving and being gracious with your own mistakes and shortcomings.

Conclusion

An important challenge to each physician and trainee is to be as serious a student of oneself as she/he is in other aspects of professional training. Most individuals are not inherently aware of the sources of "high-octane fuel" for their coping reservoir, and many assume that the drains are immutable. The knowledge and implementation of the regular practice of one's best replenishing input sources and diminishing the drains on one's coping reservoir requires a process of reflection, awareness, planning, and intention.

Examples of Positive Inputs
- Right amount of sleep on a regular basis
- Favorite types of exercise, e.g., running, yoga, dance, martial arts
- Mentoring trainees and witnessing their growth
- Connection and support from loved ones
- Processing conflict/challenging situation with mentor or trusted peer
- Other meaningful activities outside of medicine, e.g., arts, music, theater, literature
- Seeing your work make a difference
- Humor
- Flexible approach to problems
- Getting consultation on a difficult patient case
- Psychotherapy

Examples of Negative Inputs
- Anxiety that doesn't lead to a solution-oriented plan
- Fatigue especially if not addressed promptly
- Problematic, conflictual personal relationship
- Excess alcohol
- Sense of incompetence
- Sense of victimization by schedule, patient demands, flawed system
- Feeling rushed in patient care, decision-making
- Lack of connection with patients
- Secret keeping (not patient-related)
- Maintaining rigid approach to problems
- Being unwilling to admit vulnerability and imperfection

Words to the Wise
- Schedule health-promoting activities outside of medicine.
- Have an inner circle of trusted individuals with whom you can safely disclose concerns.
- Beware of irritability and losing your temper, which are often the first signs of imbalance, as well as short-term memory slips, increasing alcohol consumption, and self-prescribing.
- Embrace the truth that you do not have to do and be everything at all times.
- Be as compassionate with yourself as you would be with a loved one.

Ask Your Mentor or Colleagues
- What activity or part of life brings me the most sense of fulfillment? Can I reasonably increase the regularity or frequency of that activity? Conversely, which areas (people, activities) are the most draining?
- Are there problem/draining areas in my life that can be modified? Some things can't be removed from life completely, but can be modified. For example, a demanding administrative role you took on last year has become

increasingly challenging and certain parts may be out-side your areas of strength/expertise; are there any aspects that can be delegated or are actually not truly encompassed by that role? Another example: a demand-ing relative is part of your life, but you decide that it is possible to limit the amount or frequency of time spent with that person.

- Examine motivation: Am I doing certain activities because they seem important for academic promotion or to my mentors? Do I allow a conflictual relationship to continue because it is in fact a high-priority relationship, or out of a sense of helplessness or obligation? If it is a high-priority relationship, are there areas that could be improved via communication?

References

1. Wallace JE, Lemaire JB, Ghali WA. Physician wellness: a missing quality indicator. Lancet. 2009;374(9702):1714–21.
2. Scheurer D, McKean S, Miller J, Wetterneck T. U.S. physician satisfaction: a systematic review. J Hosp Med. 2009;4(9):560–8.
3. West CP, Huschka MM, Novotny PJ, Sloan JA, Kolars JC, Habermann TM, Shanafelt TD. Association of perceived medical errors with resident distress and empathy: a prospective longitudinal study. JAMA. 2006; 296(9):1071–8.
4. Dyrbye LN, Massie FS, Eacker A, Harper W, Power D, Durning SJ, Thomas MR, Moutier C, Satele D, Sloan JA, Shanafelt TD. Relationship between burnout and professional conduct and attitudes among US medical students: a Multi-Institutional Study. JAMA. 2010;304(11):1173–80.
5. Dyrbye LN, Thomas MR, Massie FS, Power DV, Eacker A, Harper W, Durning S, Moutier C, Szydlo DW, Novotny PJ, Sloan JA, Shanafelt TD. Burnout and suicidal ideation among US medical students. Ann Intern Med. 2008;149:334–41.
6. Schernhammer E. Taking their own lives- the high rate of physician suicide. N Eng J Med. 2005;352(24):2473–6.
7. Dunn LB, Iglewicz A, Moutier C. A conceptual model of medical student well-being: promoting resilience and preventing burnout. Acad Psychiatry. 2008;32(1):44–53.

How to Interview for a First Academic Position

4

Robert Chayer and Jon A. Lehrmann

Perhaps the most important conversation that academic clinicians ever have in their career with regard to defining their role, impact, and implications on eventual success, as well as aligning academic goals and fit within a department, is the first job interview. This critical conversation initiates what could be a lifelong relationship and defines the new faculty member's value/worth/salary. Despite the significance of this first interview, clinicians and scientists routinely receive little training or practice in preparation for it and, perhaps more important, do not learn about the process of negotiating a contract. It is true that all physicians interview for medical school and for a residency, but interviewing for the first academic medicine job is very different. In interviewing for medical school and residency, there is an assessment of overall fit from both sides of the interview, but unlike in the academic position, salary is not negotiated and there is really no negotiating over the specifics for the job. Both medical school and residency are essentially temporary arrangements. With careful negotiation, in contrast, the academic faculty member could be establishing a relationship that would serve him or her well through an entire career. This chapter introduces and discusses best practices in the interviewing process and common missteps.

J.A. Lehrmann, M.D. (✉)
Department of Psychiatry and Behavioral Medicine,
Medical College of Wisconsin, 8701 Watertown Plank Road,
Milwaukee, WI, USA
e-mail: jlehrman@mcw.edu

© Springer International Publishing Switzerland 2016
L.W. Roberts (ed.), *The Clinician Educator Guidebook*,
DOI 10.1007/978-3-319-27980-0_4

Assessment

What kind of job would be ideal? Perhaps the first and most important step in the interview process is assessing exactly what kind of job one is looking for and what other factors are critical (or merely important). The candidate should take time to focus on his or her interests, needs, and goals. It is time well spent to sit down and write out the perfect job scenario. This exercise should include at least location (city/department), inpatient/outpatient balance, on-call requirements, nature of the clinical work, variety of the patient mix, opportunities for mentorship and/or interaction with colleagues, established faculty development programs, opportunity for advancement, protected academic or research time, and stability of job or of job funding. Other factors to explore that may affect the selection of job opportunities include location or employment needs of a significant other or other family members or perhaps locating colleagues in a specific area of research interest and finding a department that has the technology or research support to help one become successful. List and rank by value/priority all of these factors. It is helpful to be clear about what exactly one is looking for. Academic jobs can vary significantly depending on the medical field, the culture of the department, and the size and flexibility of the department. The candidate needs to understand his or her strengths, weaknesses, and preferences.

Assessing a department's strengths and weaknesses and its overall fit in relation to one's own research is another critical task to accomplish during the interview. For example, mentorship is critical for academic and personal development. Does a particular department (and associated medical school) have the mentors that fit the needs one has identified, and do these individuals provide the opportunity for mentorship?

It is valuable to know some "insiders" in a target department to get the necessary information and begin to assess the department's potential "fit." Consider asking current colleagues or faculty whom they might know at the institutions of interest. It may also be beneficial to review alumni Web sites to look for former classmates who may be at an institution. A perspective from someone not actively engaged in the recruitment process may provide the most unbiased look at an institution, or at least will provide one more valuable point of reference.

Is this faculty role under consideration an internal position (a position within the department where one is currently training or working) or an external position? Each presents unique benefits and challenges. In an internal position, the candidate is already known to the department leaders and has a known reputation regarding the quality of work and work ethic. It is hoped that this will be an advantage. Additionally, there will be an increased comfort level interviewing for an internal position. Potential future managers and colleagues and the departmental culture are already well known. These factors of familiarity may have value, but they also can prevent one from taking a critical look at a job, leading to prematurely limiting options and potentially leading to not adequately preparing for a job interview (the "they already know me" factor). It is advantageous to interview at several different jobs and receive, at minimum, a couple of offers before getting serious about negotiating the particulars of a job. This practice gives leverage in negotiating (as is discussed later in the chapter) and allows the job seeker to compare best practices, benefits, and options [1]. When looking at an external position, one has a fresh start in establishing a relationship. The candidate may be courted more actively. The opportunity to build new relationships in a new department is exciting. On the other hand, one will not know the unspoken issues, and this culture in a new department may well affect one's career satisfaction. Again, if possible, it is good to have an inside connection when looking at a department.

Preparation

It is critical to do research in advance when looking at a potential job. Preparation and research should include assessing people and programs in the department. This preparation can be done by reaching out to people known to the candidate who are familiar with the department, those who are trainees from the department, or those who are current or past employees from that department [2]. Additionally, review any data available on the Internet. Learn what research and academic work the leaders in the department are doing and have done. Read some of their recent papers. Often an itinerary may be received in advance of a visit. Look up each of the faculty members who will be involved in the interview and jot down a few notes about the academic work they have done. Do some research about the current Chair and Dean, which might give some perspective as to the direction of the department and medical school. Doing this advance preparation is important from a knowledge perspective and will make an interview more productive. This process will provide some basis and background to compare the feel of the initial interview to the information garnered from the research—Do they mesh? The advance preparation will help give the candidate some confidence in interview interactions. It can also impress those conducting the interviews as they see the careful preparation as evidenced by well thought-out and informed questions.

One should definitely check the AAMC median salary for someone at the targeted faculty level in a particular region. The AAMC publishes a book of academic salaries yearly [3]. This information can provide a clearer expectation as far as what salary might be expected within academic medicine. Do not be surprised that there is a significant difference in salary between an academic position and other salaried medical positions. Understand that private practice may be more financially lucrative but leaves less opportunity for flexibility, typically involves less diversity in the work, usually lacks opportunities for mentoring, and offers fewer opportunities for sharing with colleagues.

A fairly common technique for interviewing that uses objective questions to assess faculty candidates is called performance-based interviewing or behavioral interviewing [4]. Reviewing several of these questions while formulating "best" answers from your past experiences can be very helpful. Practice interviewing with a colleague or a mentor before going to an interview to help the preparation and build confidence.

Starting the Conversation

Once you have decided that you are interested in an academic job, write a cover letter that conveys your interest and explains how your previous experience and anticipated career goals fit into the work of the department. Conveying how departmental values mesh with your values can be a good practice in this letter. (The length and level of detail of such a letter should increase with applications for higher level positions.) This cover letter should accompany an updated curriculum vitae (CV). Submitting an outdated CV shows a lack of preparation and perhaps can be read as either a lack of true interest or nonchalance about quality of work; at worst, it could be read as a sign of being disorganized or a procrastinator.

If you are interested in pursuing a job in a particular department or institution, but no jobs are currently being advertised, do not hesitate to contact department leaders. Do this significantly in advance of an anticipated change, if possible. Six months to a year in advance is typical. Often departments may not know their future situation completely and simply letting them know you are interested can get them thinking about you. Department chairmen sometimes can even create a position if they have advance notice and a candidate provides the right fit for the department. Sometimes there is unexpected turnover in a department, and contacting the chair and sending in a cover letter and CV may put a candidate in the running.

The Interview

First impressions are critical. Despite how obvious this piece of advice may be, in their academic roles the authors still do see candidates dressed in a disheveled fashion or ready for a nightclub and not the workplace. Always dress professionally, but conservatively. Be very professional and polite with all the staff, especially with the contact person and the person who is putting together the itinerary. An interview "killer" could occur if an administrative assistant tells the Chair that a candidate was rude, disrespectful, or very self-centered in interactions. Turn off cell phones and pagers before going into an interview [5]. Be very cautious should your interview include a meal where alcohol is served. It would be possible to undo all of one's careful preparation with an imprudent remark when even mildly disinhibited. If a candidate is asked about weaknesses or what is especially challenging and answers that he or she has no weaknesses, that answer can come across as the candidate having no perspective or being overly confident and can often have a negative effect. Employers want to hire faculty members who are willing to work on self-improvement and growth [6].

If you are well prepared, there really should not be any surprise questions. Expect to be asked about current job expectations and vision and how these are anticipated to change 5 years from now. Be prepared for questions about any lapses in employment history. Display a degree of flexibility throughout the interview process. Do not expect every interviewer to have read the CV and do not take it personally if they have not. Be prepared to communicate your past experience and accomplishments. It is typical to be interviewed by the Chair later in the process, and sometimes not until a second visit. Anticipate that by the time of a meeting with the Chair, there will be communication from those with whom one has spoken earlier in the process. The Chair should communicate the department's degree of interest in the candidate. Before leaving the meeting with the Chair, clarify the subsequent steps and define what the next conversation will be.

Follow-Up

Immediately after the interview, write down the pros, cons, and concerns about the position. This practice will help in days to come when comparing two jobs, or simply in preparing for a second interview. This process will facilitate clarity about questions that require follow-up. It is a best practice to promptly hand-write a personal thank-you note to each interviewer met.

Second interviews differ from first interviews in that they are more focused and they give the opportunity to clarify specifics and details about the clinical assignment, academic appointment, and expectations regarding academic work, benefits, and salary. The departmental support structure and office logistics [7] should be laid out. Benefits to be explored should include insurances (malpractice, life, disability), protected academic time, support for any further education (such as working towards a Master's degree in public health or hospital administration), book money, license fees, board exam fees, support for continuing education conferences, and so on.

Other Unique Circumstances and Sensitive Issues

When an agreement has been reached, expect that a background check will likely be a necessary part of the process. Be aware too that during the interview there are questions that are illegal and should not be asked. These include the candidate's age, marital status, membership in clubs or organizations, and citizenship [8]. Interviewers should not ask if one has been arrested or make queries about disabilities or weight or height [8]. Questions that can be asked include, Are you authorized to work in the United States? Would you be willing to relocate? Have you ever been convicted of a specific crime (named here)? Are you able to perform the essential functions of this job?

Conclusion

To summarize, the interview process is a critical part of securing academic employment. Preparation and presentation are key factors. Advanced research surrounding the department or medical school/university as well as the leaders and departmental members is essential to achieving success in the interview process. Review your interests and needs so as to be clear and direct about your priorities. To present well, it is important to dress in a professional way and have a pleasant, professional manner with all of those with whom you come into contact. Your research and the answers to questions during the interview should help you assess whether the job is the "right fit." Listen to what the department needs and suggest how you will be a clear asset and meet its needs. The end result of this process should be the offer of a position that holds anticipation and excitement for both the individual and for the institution and ideally, the beginning of a fruitful and satisfying academic career.

Words to the Wise
- Know the academic work of the Chair and key faculty members.
- Utilize professional behavior and appearance.
- Anticipate and practice writing out answers to Performance-Based Inter viewing questions.
- Send thank-yous to each interviewer.

Ask Your Mentor or Colleagues
- What do you feel would be the best fit for me in an academic job?
- What do you see as my strengths and weaknesses, and what would be the best way to convey and frame them in an interview?
- Would you be willing to practice a "mock" job interview with me?

References

1. Fisher R, Ury WL, Patton B. Getting to yes: negotiating agreement without giving in. New York, NY: Houghton Mifflin Harcourt; 1991.
2. Dungy CI, DeWitt TG, Nelson KG. Securing a faculty position: a practical guide for residents, fellows, junior faculty, and their mentors. Ambul Pediatr. 2005;5:235–9.
3. Association of American Medical Colleges (AAMC) report on medical school faculty salaries, 2009–2010.
4. United States Veterans Affairs: Performance based interviewing (PBI) home. http://www.va.gov/pbi. Accessed 21 Dec 2011.
5. Tufts University: Interviewing skills. http://www.tufts.edu/med/about/student-resources/careerservices/resources/interviewing.html. Accessed 21 Dec 2011.
6. Kaplan R. Handling illegal questions [Jobweb Web site]. http://www.jobweb.com/resources/library/Interviews/Handling_Illegal_46_02htm. Accessed Oct 2011.
7. Roberts LW, Hilty D, editors. Handbook of career development in academic psychiatry and behavioral sciences: interviewing for an academic position. Washington, DC: American Psychiatric Press; 2006. p. 61–8.
8. Scrignoli T. "How to ace the job interview". American College of Physicians Website Marketing yourself section: www.acponline.org/residents_fellows/career_counseling/guidance.htm. Oct 2010. Career guide for residents pdf.

How to Evaluate a Letter of Offer or Contract

5

Andrew Norton

The letter of offer or contract represents the official intent of a hiring institution toward a candidate. The process of making a good decision regarding any offer starts long before the candidate receives the document. Decisions are made within the broad context of one's cumulative life experiences, education, work experiences, influences of family and mentors, travel and cultural experiences, and even spiritual and religious background. All of these factors will help frame the priorities that the academic physician will bring to the decision-making process. The candidate must recognize that he or she is often influenced by more immediate experiences, potentially to the detriment of seeing things from a broader perspective. If experiences in his or her most recent job or during a just-completed residency or fellowship were all that the candidate were considering at this phase, the candidate would likely not make the most informed decision. Work–life balance, income expectations, a blended career, or a more focused career are all examples of characteristics of jobs that will have to be

A. Norton, M.D. (✉)
Department of Clinical Medicine, Medical College of Wisconsin,
9200 W. Wisconsin Ave, Milwaukee, WI, USA
e-mail: anorton@mcw.edu

© Springer International Publishing Switzerland 2016
L.W. Roberts (ed.), *The Clinician Educator Guidebook*,
DOI 10.1007/978-3-319-27980-0_5

considered in this phase. The clearer these priorities are for the candidate, the higher the likelihood that a good decision will be made. Having clarity on these issues helps not only during this process but also throughout one's career. These priorities can be a touchstone to which the academic physician returns during the critical phases throughout his or her career.

Using the Search Process to Prepare for Reviewing a Letter of Offer or Contract

Throughout the process of searching for, interviewing for, and considering any new position, the candidate must prepare for the next phase of the job acquisition process, namely, the review and negotiation of a letter of offer or contract. Although the letter of offer is the official declaration of intent by the hiring institution, the candidate should be well along the mental process of deciding whether that institution would be a good fit at the time that he or she receives the letter. The goal of any recruitment process is for both parties, the candidate and the hiring institution, to find the best match. The candidate's due diligence during the interview and negotiation process will go a long way to ensuring a good fit. By the time the candidate receives a letter of offer, he or she should have a basic understanding of the offering institution, its organizational structure, its employment environment, and the candidate's general role within the organization. Thoughtfully accumulating specific employment-related information throughout the interview process will facilitate this phase. A 2×2 decision grid listing the institutions that one is considering and some key characteristics is an example of a simple tool to use throughout the interview process. Whether or not this is one's first experience with a letter of offer, this phase of the job selection process is important and warrants thoughtful and deliberate effort, which could be shortchanged in the enthusiasm to close the deal.

Before beginning the interview process, the candidate would benefit from meeting with 2–3 senior faculty members or mentors to receive their input on the interview process, job characteristics, employment models, and so on. Ideally these advisors would have insight into the candidate's skills and career aspirations, so their advice would be specifically tailored to the circumstances. If one is working with a recruitment firm, utilize its expertise in outlining the key characteristics of the institutions being considered. The more a candidate knows about an institution before the interview, the more information the candidate will glean about the institution during the interview. Specific questions, prepared in advance, can increase one's confidence that he or she has adequate information available in the deliberation phase of the hiring process. The candidate will find it much easier to gather information about an institution during his or her site visits, where the opportunities, both structured and spontaneous, are numerous. Trying to find that information after the interview is more challenging. The decision whether one would use legal counsel to review the contract should really be made before one starts the process. If the candidate decides to use legal counsel, that person should be hired and met with before the interview process begins. The legal counsel's perspectives will help prepare the candidate to get even more out of the interview. Be sure to hire an attorney with considerable health care experience, who knows the unique issues related to health care institutions and physician employment and compensation.

Use the entire interview process to prepare for reviewing a letter of offer. Careful assessments of one's personal goals, accumulation of external input from experts, careful accumulation of information to compare and contrast opportunities, and thoughtful discussions about life goals with people about whom one cares are all essential elements of the process. Preparation of checklists and decision grids will make the process easier. Recognize that the recruitment process is often overlapping and not in sync between interviews, second visits, and offers, which makes clearly defining key decision criteria all the more important. The candidate may find that his or her schedule is full and time limited at the critical phase of the process of making a final decision of whether to accept a job offer. While the interview process itself will help in creating some clarity, the candidate should not use the interview process alone in decision making. Often there will not be adequate time for deliberate introspection when one is considering more than one job offer, each with its own time limit for a yes/no response.

Be sure to ask for an official employment handbook at the time of the initial interview. Often these are not offered during the first interview without special request. This information can be invaluable and easily perused during the trip back home. During this immediate post-interview period, take the time to review any materials that were obtained during the interview, add information to the decision grid, and develop specific follow-up questions that would be answered during a second interview or letter of offer review. This is also the time to jot down the key characteristics of the institution, both positive and negative, which will serve as a reference for subsequent site visits and discussions with leaders at the institution.

The use of social media in the recruitment process is still in its infancy. Institutional Web sites can certainly provide basic information. Web-based services such as LinkedIn and Monster may provide networking opportunities, content resources, answers to FAQs, and so on, but the use of such sites as an active part of the recruitment process is unlikely. Be aware that prospective employers can access any personal information available on the Internet.

Once the Offer Is Made

You just got off the phone. A verbal offer has been made which you have accepted pending the review of a letter of offer or contract. You are excited, enthusiastic about the new position, and cannot wait to get started. However, it is important to take adequate time during this phase to be sure that you understand all the elements of the employment agreement. The signed letter of offer or contract as well as any referenced employee handbooks, codes of conduct, and standards of care all make up the legally binding employment agreement and trump any verbal offers or commitments made during the recruitment process.

During the negotiation phase, keep the lines of communication with the hiring chair or chief open and active. There is often a lag between the time that the verbal offer is made and the written letter of agreement/contract and referenced employee handbook materials are received. Use this window of time to send a letter to your likely new boss that, in your words, describes what you think the job elements and expectations are. This represents an opportunity for you to communicate what you thought you heard as it relates to the job elements and expectations and what you think is most important. You should highlight the key deliverables that you expect to be covered in your written contract or letter of offer. Taking this proactive step will often shorten the negotiation process and bring clarity to key elements of the job opportunity.

Recognize that there will be negotiable and nonnegotiable components of the letter of offer or contract. Leaders in larger institutions may have less ability to negotiate certain components of the contract. An important question is to clarify what components of the letter of offer or contract are negotiable. If you have engaged an attorney, set up time now to sit down and review the letter of offer or contract.

The Contract/Letter of Offer

Each institution will have its own format to its written employment agreement. It may be a formal contract or it may be a letter of offer. Either will be supplemented with legally binding amendments as articulated in employee handbooks or like vehicles. There is no legal difference between a written contract and a letter of agreement; both carry the weight of a formal contract. The amount of detail in these documents will vary. Some may not have enough specificity and will require a request for further detail and specifics in writing. Some of these documents will have been developed at a central institutional contracts-and-human-resources level; others will be created at the hiring-department level. What is critical is whether you feel you have adequate detail in these documents for the purposes of negotiation and ultimately acceptance of the offer.

The key components of the letter of offer/contract include terms, terminations, and restrictive covenants; academic rank; duties and responsibilities; and compensation. Each is discussed in turn in the subsequent text.

Terms, Terminations, and Restrictive Covenants

Most academic contracts are annual and self-renewing on the basis of reasonable performance. What is critical to understand are the elements of performance assessment and the bilateral obligations for contract termination. Causes for termination are typically outlined in the employee handbook. Often not articulated in adequate detail are the review process, due process obligations, and access to fair hearing components. Resignation by the employee typically will require 3–6 months of advance notification to allow for transfer of patient care and academic and research obligations. There can be a financial penalty for inadequate notice for the costs of this responsibility transfer. Many contracts and employment relationships include a process by which the institution can initiate a nonrenewal or a termination process outside of a grievance process, such as in the form of a nonrenewal clause in the contract typically with 1-year notice. This process would be used if a faculty member had performed adequately but was not felt to be a good fit for a long-term faculty position. Academic rank, tenure, and specific clauses in individual contracts may affect the institution's latitude in such a nonrenewal process. As a result, many medical centers do not have severance agreements, although these can be negotiated in individual circumstances.

Employment agreements are commonly applied to all new faculty members and are used to protect the business interests of the hiring academic institution while the faculty member is employed or after the employment relationship ends. Such agreements usually have three components: a confidentiality provision, a nonsolicitation clause, and a restrictive covenant. The confidentiality provision prevents postemployment solicitation of other employees and/or patients, and the restrictive covenant outlines restrictions on postemployment competition with the academic center. Understanding these agreements in detail is critical, and legal authorities feel that they are enforceable if reasonable.

Although considering termination and restrictive covenant issues in the excitement of starting a new job can feel uncomfortable—as if one were anticipating a negative outcome—the reality of these issues warrants adequate review and understanding before signing a contract—not when faced with the need to use such components.

Academic Rank

The academic rank that the department chair or division chief will recommend on a candidate's appointment to the faculty will not typically be a point of contention or negotiation, especially for one's initial faculty position. However, in the case of an academic physician making a midcareer position change, it will be important to clarify academic rank criteria at the new institution and to come to an agreement with the hiring chair or chief as to the academic rank for which the candidate will be recommended. In most institutions, the final decision will be made by the rank and tenure committee, notwithstanding the proposed academic rank by the hiring chair or chief. If maintaining one's current rank or moving up an academic rank is a critical criteria in the selection of a new position, be sure to raise that issue during the recruitment process.

Duties and Responsibilities

The duties and responsibilities section is the section of the letter of offer or contract in which the candidate should expect and request the most detail. As previously recommended, the candidate can facilitate this section by submitting a letter to the hiring official with a detailed listing of the candidate's understanding of the duties and responsibilities. Specifics matter. For example, the distribution of work effort should be defined, including both floor and ceiling, as well as expectations regarding average work hours (e.g., no less than 20 % time will be spent in clinical care; not to exceed 50 % of an average work week of 55 h).

The more common components of duties and responsibilities will include the following items:

- Distribution of work effort: Clinical, educational, research, administrative, academic service (membership on committees), and community service. Who determines this, what influence the candidate has on it, and the intervals between reallocations should be determined.
- Lines of communication and authority: Clarify with the division chief or department chair who specifically is one's superior

and to whom one must account for job responsibilities in each of these areas. Although most often one will be accountable to the division chief or department chair, be aware of comanagement environments such as clinics that have medical directors; research laboratories and core laboratories that have directors; and hospital services in which responsibility is shared with hospital directors. Each of these could create confusion regarding time allocations, measurement of accountabilities, and resource allocations.

• Measurement of performance: For academic clinicians, this could include clinical productivity, clinical outcomes, patient satisfaction, clinical utilization, and expense management (expense/RVU). For researchers, typical measures would include obtaining grant support, with timelines and financial amounts explicitly defined; publications; participation in national study groups; evaluations from postdoctoral students; and participation in academic service. For educators, measurements would include learner evaluations, publications, and curriculum development. Knowing if any of these measures of performance are linked to compensation or incentives would be critical. Clear understanding of who determines performance measures, who does the evaluations, and how often performance measures are reviewed and updated should be outlined.

• Infrastructure and support expectations: These will differ depending on the clinical, research, administrative, or educational focus of the candidate, but they need to be spelled out in adequate detail, including office, lab, or clinical space; support staff (administrative, research, or clinical); and technical support, including IT. For clinicians, issues such as call, vacation, or illness coverage should be understood. Finding out after starting that one's clinical workload goes up by 50 % because a clinical colleague broke a hip and needed surgery can be an unexpected and unwelcome surprise. Adequate support staff in the clinical environment is as critical as adequate lab space and research associate to the researcher to maximize efficiency, productivity, compensation, and satisfaction. Check if clinic or lab overhead is linked to compensation.

Compensation

Compensation includes base salary, incentives, and bonuses. Compensation strategies will vary depending on the academic role in the institution. Common forms of compensation include the following:

- Fixed salary: The benefit is predictability. The downside for the hiring institution is accountability for performance and productivity. The downside for the faculty member is the lack of incentives or bonuses based on exceptional performance.
- Base salary with a variable component: This increasingly common compensation method blends a level of predictability with the ability to set performance-based metrics that link to compensation, including productivity, patient satisfaction, clinical outcomes, and expense management.
- Production-based compensation based on total clinical collections minus a fixed expense rate.

Be sure to understand the formulas by which incentives and bonuses are determined, timelines for payout, and who is in charge of setting the incentives and determining the metrics and how often they are adjusted. National benchmarks for salaries and benefits can be obtained from groups such as the Association of American Medical Colleges (AAMC) and the Medical Group Management Association (MGMA).

There are a number of reimbursements and fees that should be spelled out in the letter of offer or contract. Fees could include parking fees, use of campus services such as core labs, video services, and data analysis/statistical support. Reimbursement for items such as computer and IT support, practice-related expenses such as license fees and professional association dues, work-related travel, continuing medical education, and professional society expenses should be explained. These are typically negotiable. Transition expenses including relocation expenses, both personal and research lab related, should be negotiated.

If it is possible that the candidate may generate intellectual property through his or her academic work, he or she should fully understand the intellectual property policies of the hiring institution—clearly, an area that requires special expertise. The institution may, however, consider this policy a nonnegotiable area of the employment relationship.

Employee Handbooks

Employee handbooks are a key component of the overall employment package and should be carefully reviewed. The handbook will be referenced in the letter of offer or contract and is considered a binding part of the agreement between hiring institution and the faculty member. The handbook will be developed at the institutional level, and the human resources department should be used for questions for clarification. If the handbook is obtained during the interview visit, the candidate will have time to review it in detail and identify areas for clarification during subsequent visits or during the contract negotiation phase.

Key components of the handbook are as follows:

- Health insurance
- Wellness incentives, including health club discounts
- Life insurance
- Disability, both short- and long-term
- Malpractice insurance
- Vacation and sick time benefits
- Retirement plan options, including times of vesting
- Childcare provisions
- Employer policies and procedures

It is worth spending a little time reviewing the key components of the institution's policies and procedures on such diverse issues as grievance and due process, Health Insurance Portability and Accountability Act (HIPAA) information and other confidentiality agreements, and codes of conduct or related professional behavioral policies. The academic physician will be held to the standards, and it is the appropriate expectation of the hiring institution that the candidate be aware of them, understand them, and apply them in the work environment.

It is often these key elements of an employment relationship that are least understood by the department chair or chief who will be guiding the candidate through the recruitment process. Department administrators and members of the central human resources office of the institution are excellent resources on the specifics of the employment relationship. Asking for a scheduled time with a human resources representative as part of the interview process will be helpful in one's final review of the contract or letter of offer.

Finally, a few comments on whether to obtain legal advice. Contractual language may be nuanced. Lawyers will help with important clarifications and legal elements of the contract or letter of offer. When is it appropriate to hire a contract lawyer? It depends on the complexity and duration of the contract, issues such as employment agreements that include restrictive covenants and control over intellectual property, and the legal expertise and comfort of the physician.

Words to the Wise
- Preparation matters. Spending time understanding one's personal and career objectives, key components of job satisfaction, and critical employment requirements before beginning the interview process is important.
- Categorize the key components of employment (e.g., work responsibilities, benefits, compensation, call coverage) and keep a comparison grid that allows one to look at the various opportunities in a systematic and organized way.
- Once given a verbal offer, and before receiving a formal letter of offer, prepare and send a written summary of the job and its key elements as one understands it, which will help set a framework for the formal letter of offer and negotiations of key points.
- Spend time with the employee handbook and understand key areas of basic employee benefits (e.g., health insurance, disability insurance, malpractice coverage).
- Be willing to negotiate key elements and to ask for clarification in writing of key elements such as compensation, distribution of work effort, call coverage, and bonus programs.

Ask Your Mentor or Colleagues
- What is the greatest lesson learned from your own recruit-ment and employment experiences?
- What components of your employment agreement do you wish you had had a better understanding of during the recruitment process? What effect has that had on your career, finances, and/or satisfaction?
- What is the one thing you wish you had known in advance of your first job search that you would like me to know?
- Can you recommend specific resources into which I should tap?

Appendix: Sample Letter of Offer

[Date]

Dear Dr.:-----------------

We are pleased to extend to you an offer of appointment to the full-time faculty in the Department of-----------------------, anticipated to commence on------------------.

Your appointment will be proposed at the rank of Assistant Professor. Policies governing faculty appointments are contained in the enclosed *Information for Faculty* handbook.

Your initial contributions to college and departmental missions in the areas of patient care, teaching, research, and administration/service will be as follows:-----------------------
--.

Patient care: Your primary clinical assignment will be----------------. In addition to this inpatient work, you will devote approximately six (6) hours per week to the Department's------------Program----------------directed by------------------. You will be expected to participate in the on call rotation, with duties consistent with your team members. We anticipate this will be--------------------.

Teaching: In your role, you will be expected to participate in the multidisciplinary educational programs of the Department, to include---------.

Research: In your role, you will be expected to collaborate with faculty involved in clinical trials and other clinical research protocols on average for four (4) hours per week.

Administration/Service: You will be expected to participate, to the extent that you may be reasonably called upon, in administrative and/or service functions of the Department and the Medical School.

Your salary for the -------- academic year will be at the annual rate of $ --------. Thereafter, your compensation will be reviewed at least annually, and sources of funding and FTE allocations may change that may affect your salary.

The Department will cover the registration fee for the--------board certification examination should you choose to take it. We encourage you to do so. This reimbursement may be considered taxable income to you.

Faculty Practice Plan; Clinical Services Agreement; Compliance with Medicare and Medicaid Laws and Regulations; Mandatory Education: You will become a member of the------------and be subject to its rules and the Faculty Practice Plan. You will also be required to enter into a Clinical Services Agreement and Restrictive Covenant with--------
----and to comply with and attend educational sessions on Medicare and Medicaid laws and regulations. All patient care performed by you will be billed through the Faculty Practice Plan, and the resulting income will be the property of-------------------. A Faculty Practice Plan billing number will be issued to you prior to your engaging in any patient care activities.

The-----------------has adopted a Code of Conduct, a copy of which is enclosed. As a condition of employment, you must acknowledge that you have received, read, and understood the Code of Conduct. The acknowledgement form is also enclosed and must be signed and returned.

Additional Conditions of Appointment. This offer of appointment is also subject to the following:

1.   Your agreement to comply with the bylaws, policies, and procedures of------------
---, including the *Information for Faculty* handbook, and the Code of Conduct;
2.   Your obtaining and maintaining an unlimited----------------medical license and DEA registration;
3.   Your acceptance by the-----------------for professional liability (malpractice) insurance coverage;
4.   Your obtaining and maintaining medical staff membership and clinical privileges at the hospital(s) where you will be assigned;
5.   Your eligibility to participate in the Medicare and Medicaid programs, and your ability to be credentialed for treatment of managed care patients; and----------------
--.

Your anticipated start date is dependent on the satisfaction of all conditions specified in this letter. Because the process is time sensitive, it is important that you complete and return all required forms promptly. If you accept the terms and conditions of the appointment contained in this letter of offer, please sign and return one copy of the letter within the next two weeks, accompanied by the Code of Conduct acknowledgement form, Clinical Services Agreement, Professional Liability Self-Insurance Questionnaire, and Credentialing Application completed according to the enclosed instructions.

Upon receipt of your signed acceptance of this offer and other required materials, and the satisfaction of all other conditions of appointment, we will forward our recommendations to our Dean's office for consideration.

Very truly yours,

Chair,

Department of----------------
       Dean and Executive Vice President

Enclosures

ACCEPTANCE OF OFFER OF APPOINTMENT
I accept the offer of appointment described in this letter subject to all its terms and conditions.

Signature

Print name: ------------------------

Date: ------------------------

How to Give a Lecture

6

Sallie G. DeGolia

The lecture is alive and well within medical education despite the increased emphasis over decades on small-group teaching and problem-based learning [1, 2]. All US and Canadian medical schools are still using lecture formats as an important teaching vehicle in at least the first 2 years of medical school [3]. Furthermore, the "*See One, Do One, Teach One*" classical approach to medical education also continues to thrive when it comes to lecturing. Most educators learn how to lecture by having experienced a lecture as students rather than by participating in any professional development workshop or training [4, 5]. But being an expert of content does not necessarily translate into being a proficient lecturer. With increasing demands from the Accreditation Council for Graduate Medical Education (ACGME) for higher standards of accountability for student learning, faculty seek to improve educational methods. This chapter serves as a guide to help make the lecture a more efficient and effective learning tool.

S.G. DeGolia, M.P.H., M.D. (✉)
Department of Psychiatry and Behavioral Sciences,
Stanford University Hospital and Clinics, 401 Quarry Road,
Stanford, CA, USA
e-mail: degolia@stanford.edu

© Springer International Publishing Switzerland 2016
L.W. Roberts (ed.), *The Clinician Educator Guidebook*,
DOI 10.1007/978-3-319-27980-0_6

Purpose of the Lecture

Lecturing is an economical and efficient method of delivering information to a large group of learners. It may expose learners to a new subject or alternative perspectives, model a way of thinking, challenge accepted beliefs and attitudes, promote thought, deepen understanding, stimulate further learning, provide a way to present up-to-date material not available in print, and even serve a social function [6–8].

Learning Theories

By designing lectures with adult learning concepts and new approaches to teaching and learning in mind, the academic faculty member can make the lecture a valuable learning experience. Adult learners generally can be characterized as being self-directed and motivated, relying upon their previous experience to enhance their learning, needing intellectual justification for learning specific topics, and wanting evidence to explain how learning a given content area will contribute to their professional understanding and how they might apply it in the future. Adult learners also want to apply their new knowledge immediately in solving problems and receive feedback on their progress [9].

In an attempt to achieve meaningful or deep learning, students must focus on understanding the content instead of memorizing facts and concepts. Striving to understand the new knowledge as a coherent whole rather than a set of disparate facts leads to meaningful learning. This type of learning can be distinguished from surface learning, which focuses on excessive amounts of material and memorization and uses assessment methods that emphasize recall and provide little or inadequate feedback. Searching for clues of what should be learned instead of focusing on understanding the material results in superficial learning. Therefore, by helping students build relationships and connections with existing knowledge, providing opportunities for students to actively engage with the material through various teaching modalities, and encouraging long-term involvement with the topic, deep learning can take place.

The prerequisites of meaningful learning include pre-understanding, the relevant context for the material, and encouraging activity [8]. In order to integrate new knowledge into the learner's awareness as a meaningful whole, learners must relate this new information to what the learner already knows or thinks of a situation or phenomenon—the preexisting knowledge. The learner also must appreciate the relevance and importance of the content; this will help motivate the student to learn the content. The learner must be an active participant in the learning process in order to integrate the knowledge in a meaningful way.

Furthermore, material transmitted must be perceived, attended to, and placed in short- and long-term memory. What learners choose to perceive is determined by what they already know, what interests them, and their levels of attention and arousal, among other things. New information received by the learner is filtered and stored in short-term memory. If this information is not immediately transferred to long-term memory, it will be forgotten [10]. If the preexisting knowledge has been activated and is closely related to the new incoming material, this new information will be more readily received by the long-term memory. Therefore, the lecture must be interesting, relevant, and somewhat associated to the preexisting knowledge such that learners will attend to it and absorb the material.

Steps to Creating the Effective Lecture

Preparation

So how does one develop an effective lecture? Careful preparation and organization, audiovisual aids, attention to performance behaviors, and evaluation are critical components of ensuring an effective lecture. Do not overlook the preliminary planning: knowing the context in which you will present your lecture, the intended audience, and your content is pivotal to the preparation.

Know the context. Consider the context in which you are lecturing. What is the purpose of the overall program? How does your lecture relate to the overall curricular plan? What type of presentation is expected? Are you providing a presentation in a course sequence or is it a stand-alone, one-time presentation? What are the allotted time frame or facilities available to you?

Know your audience. To whom are you delivering this content? Know your learners' existing knowledge base and their cognitive structure. Where are they in terms of their professional development and knowledge regarding the topic you plan to present? What seems to interest your learners? Why do the learners need to learn this content? Making content relevant to this particular group of learners will help motivate them to learn and value what you are presenting.

Know your content. Select the content to be delivered. Do not rely on one text but synthesize your content from a variety of materials. Consider not only the knowledge component of your material but also aspects relating to skills and attitudes where appropriate. On the basis of who your learners are, determine what parts of the material are interesting and critically important to learn. Limit the amount of material to be covered.

Organization

Once you have identified the appropriate content with your learners' characteristics and the context in mind, you are ready to organize your content. The overall rule of thumb is *Say what you are going to say, say it, then say it again.* Start with developing clear, specific, learner-focused learning objectives. Allot enough time for each objective to promote optimal organization of your presentation.

Assemble a coherent framework for your content from which you can explain the material. This framework can be accomplished in a variety of ways but two common approaches include the *hierarchical and chaining* [6]. The classical hierarchy is the commonest and simplest format. It is particularly useful for inexperienced lecturers. Start with a unifying topic with subgroups branching out in a parallel manner. Subpoints from the subgroups are then further divided into more detail. Because the average number of items that can be held in short-term memory is about seven, do not overload the learner with details but allow plenty of time for processing of the information [11]. Although the classical hierarchy is an effective way to present facts, the downside is that it can be a rather rigid schema because facts are pre-grouped.

Another related schema is using the problem-centered approach, where an identified problem is presented followed by outlining associated, alternative solutions or hypotheses that are based on the evidence. The evidence is used to support the hypotheses or solutions through a process of reasoning instead of relationships of classification, as used in the hierarchical model. This problem-centered approach tends to stimulate learner interest. The disadvantage is that it can be challenging, because it assumes learners' preexisting knowledge and requires a clear understanding of the initial problem.

The second major organizational approach is *chaining*. This approach connects ideas in time while linking them through the use of reasoning. The story-telling method, a type of chaining, describes content by employing a beginning, middle, and end and is typically presented in a conversational manner. Students tend to listen more attentively and with interest when a story-telling approach is utilized.

Other suggested organizational schemas include the following:

- *Cause and Effect.* Events are described and explained by reference to their origins.
- *Pro–Con or Compare–Contrast.* Present two sides of a given problem.
- *Ascending–Descending.* Arrange topics in relation to their importance, familiarity, or complexity to the overall topic from most to least.
- *Phenomena/Examples to Theory.* Present the phenomena or examples first followed by the theory to explain them.
- *Concepts–Application.* Present concepts and then the application in which they are applied.

By providing a conceptual framework for understanding the material to be presented, the lecturer allows learners to follow the presentation and identify the critical ideas. Structure the information in a logical fashion. Do not overload the lecture with information because time will be needed for interactive activities.

Beginning

Key components in the introduction phase of the lecture involve establishing a positive learning environment, stating the learning objectives, capturing the attention of the audience, and generating interest for the topic at hand.

Establish a positive learning environment. Creating an open and supportive atmosphere where learners are encouraged to actively participate is critical to enhancing learning [12]. Attempt to minimize any stress within this environment at the outset: Check the room temperature and potential for interruptions, verify adequate lighting and visual accessibility, ensure adequate space for learner materials, check technology requirements and operation, and alert learners to silence any cell phones or pagers. Also, where possible, the lecturer might use learner names. Always encourage and reinforce participation, show enthusiasm for the topic and learners, and be respectful.

State learning objectives and previews. At the very start, establish what the learner is expected to learn by the end of the lecture by stating learner objectives. These should be described as clear, specific, observable, and measurable learner behaviors. For example, "The learner will be able to compare and contrast the mechanisms of action of the various antihypertensive medications" by the end of the lecture. These objectives can be written on the board or presented on a slide. The objectives may be presented in the form of questions to challenge and evoke the learner's curiosity. Explain why these learning objectives are important for the learner to master.

Furthermore, provide a preview of the lecture by outlining its structure in terms of main topics, issues, and theories. If the lecture is part of a series, place the lecture in context by linking the material to earlier sessions. This preview serves to focus your learners on key points of the lecture and helps them organize and anticipate what will be happening throughout the lecture [13]. Refer to this outline periodically to reorient the learners.

Gain the attention and interest of your audience. Generating interest is essential in a presentation if you want your learners to attend to what you are presenting. This interest influences students' attitudes toward a subject and promotes learning [14].

Depending on the size of your audience, you can start off the lecture with an icebreaker to relax the participants as well as yourself. For example, have people introduce themselves and tell a little about their background as it might relate to the topic, identifying themselves with their name and a one-word self-description or, if grouped at tables, identifying something in common with the other learners.

There are many ways to gain the learner's attention for the topic. Useful techniques may include presenting a clinical or humorous anecdote that is relevant to the learners, asking a provocative question or using a dramatic contrast, or giving a short questionnaire or demonstration. Even showing a short video may be of value. Vary what you use to open the lecture, because repetition leads to less effect over time.

Assuming a narrative mode of explaining also may build interest. Mixing explanatory modes by beginning with the narrative or story-telling approach and then inserting anecdotes where appropriate and ending with a conceptual summary is a particularly effective way to generate interest and understanding [10]. Furthermore, behavioral dimensions including warmth, enthusiasm, conversational style, energy, and charisma will also increase a learner's interest and attention to the topic.

Build on previous experience. Attempt to stimulate the learners to recall previous learning and capabilities. Activating a learner's preexisting knowledge linked to the new material will help facilitate the integration of the new content into the preexisting knowledge, which serves to enhance retention. Some examples include stating, "You all know about …" or using an advance organizer, a technique where information is presented before learning and can be used by the learner to organize and interpret new, incoming material [15]. The advance organizer typically is presented at a more abstract level than the content of the lecture and serves to bridge the gap from what the learner already knows and what the learner needs to know.

Middle

Once the audience is primed to receive the new information, the lecturer is ready to deliver the body of the talk. For a 50-min lecture, no more than 3–5 main points should be presented so that learners can manage the information. Focus on important, needed, and interesting content, with each point addressing the main theme in some way. Emphasize principles and rules with a few details. Too many details are difficult to remember and tend to interfere with understanding [6].

Clarify ideas by using cases, examples, or anecdotes. In addition, pausing every 12–15 min for students to process the information or engaging the learners in an active manner increases learning. Vary the methods of explanation (examples, interactive tasks, questions, demonstrations, video clips, etc.) to maintain audience attention and stimulation.

Clarity

Several strategies can be employed to optimize clarity, such as the following:

- Provide a clear structure.
- Avoid vague terms.
- Define new terms.
- Emphasize key points.
- Use images to guide the learner.
- Name and label various parts and point precisely at diagrams.
- Offer examples, metaphors, and analogies.
- Use repetition.
- Paraphrase the key points.
- Employ transitions.
- Adequately answer learner questions.

Examples and supporting materials can be added to each main point. Examples tie theory to reality and relate concepts to the concrete. Appropriate examples and anecdotes can make material meaningful; however, keep them brief. Examples and analogies also can serve to link the structure of the topic to the learner's cognitive structure. The order in which examples are presented is important. If content is new to the learners, an effective way to link known information to new knowledge is to first explain this material through several examples followed by a definition or generalization. If the material is relatively familiar to the audience, start with stating the principle followed by examples. This helps restructure existing knowledge [16].

Other strategies to promote clarity include explaining relationships in material by comparing and contrasting, using analogies, and encouraging students to develop concept maps. Responding adequately to learners' questions also helps to promote clarity in the learners' minds. Using structuring moves such as enumerating and employing clear transitional phrases (e.g., "next," "let's move on to," "now we will consider…") to move from one subtopic to another and summarizing key points at each section of an explanation help the learner follow the presentation and stay focused.

Use periodic summaries for longer lectures and refer back to the learning objectives to remind learners where they are in the lecture. Periodic reviews help learners consolidate the information and help those who momentarily drift off to return to the flow of the presentation.

Other important tips to consider regarding clarity involve speaking clearly, using pauses effectively, and not speaking too fast.

Interactive Techniques

Incorporating interactive techniques into a lecture allows learners to actively engage with the new material by practicing their cognitive skills. Though this approach may seem formidable in a large lecture hall, several strategies have been described in the literature. Interactive strategies serve to generate interest among learners, allow learners to apply the new knowledge and check their understanding, and also serve to renew a waning attention span among the participants. Learner attention tends to decrease significantly after 20 min into a lecture and only picks up right before the end of a lecture [17]. Interactive techniques may serve to link one section of a lecture to another. Furthermore, students tend to learn better by participating in interactive learning environments while enjoying the social interactions [18]. Students find collaboration groups fun, nonthreatening, and dynamic. Such strategies also can result in increased attendance and an increased desire to participate in discussions. Interactive groups also serve to shift the learning onus from the teacher to the learner and provide the teacher important information about the learners' understanding of the material being taught. Some examples of interactive strategies include questioning, buzz groups or cooperative groups, and audience response systems. These will be described in greater detail in the subsequent text.

Questioning: The tried-and-true, non-technological approach to engage students is asking questions. Questions can be directed to individual students, small groups, or the entire group. Attempt to ask higher order questions, such as synthesis–analysis types, as opposed to recall questions. Allow at least 3–5 s of wait time for students to formulate their responses. Using student names as well as providing positive reinforcement when students respond can be a powerful motivator and tend to encourage more participation.

Allowing students to ask questions is also important. Repeat any question and answer so that all students can benefit from the discussion (repetition also gives the lecturer time to think about the question). Take your time, if needed, to find answers to questions; this shows that you value the learner's education. Responding to a student's question can also provide clarity and feedback to the student and topic.

If asking a question to the class or an individual and expecting a verbal response seems too cumbersome, consider asking students to answer a question on a piece of paper, which promotes engagement with the new material and, if the answers are reviewed, can inform the lecturer how well the material has been explained.

Buzz Groups or Cooperative Groups: Invite the class to break into groups of 3–4 students to consider a question or a problem to solve, develop an example of a concept, or formulate a question about something not understood from the preceding part of the lecture. After a few minutes of discussion, a group-selected leader can present the group's results to the class, or the teacher can summarize comments or a solution on a whiteboard. Not only do the learners actively engage with the content, but also they receive feedback from both peers and the teacher.

Audience Response Systems: Students enjoy using an audience response system [19, 20], although the data are mixed regarding its effect on knowledge retention [19–22]. The system tends to encourage more active participation and more honest responses as it preserves students' anonymity [19]. The instructor can stop periodically throughout the lecture to question the learners and track individual and/or group responses. This immediate feedback allows learners to gauge how well they understand the material while informing the instructor how effective his or her explanation has been and whether the instructor needs to rephrase or repeat concepts. This technology provides another way to highlight key points being delivered.

Handouts and Notes: Several different types of handouts are possible, but in general, the larger the audience, the more important the handouts are. Handouts can include a one-page outline of key points, interactive skeletal notes requiring completion during the lecture, complex diagrams or references, transcripts of the lecture, or exercises to be used during the lecture.

Interactive or guided notes require students to actively engage in lecture material. They improve accuracy and efficiency of note taking and increase retention of content [23]. In general, the acts of taking and reviewing notes improve recall [6]. By providing complete or skeletal lecture slides, students have the accurate information and do not need to focus on copying words. Instead, learners are encouraged to use higher order skills such as synthesis and comparing and contrasting material.

Handouts should reflect the purpose and structure of the presentation. Prepare the handouts from the audience's perspective and with their future use in mind [24]. Engage the learner by providing empty spaces to write key facts, concepts, and/or relationships during the lecture or a list of questions to be discussed during class. If the handout is made available before the class, the learner has the chance to preview the content.

Worksheets to be completed after the presentation may include printouts of abbreviated slides, incomplete diagrams, exercises with fill-in-the blanks, or incomplete lists of advantages or disadvantages of a topic outlined. Other handouts to be distributed to learners might include related resources, Internet sites, and articles.

Other Techniques: Several other techniques have also been employed to encourage learners to engage actively with the lecture content:

- Identify Main Concepts: The lecturer instructs the students at the beginning to make notes of key concepts as they move through the lecture and present them at the end.
- Concept Maps: Ask learners to develop concept maps following the lecture to actively create conceptual links from the lecture material. The concept maps are constructed by connecting individual terms by lines that indicate the relationship between each set of connected terms. Most of the terms in a concept map have multiple connections. Developing a concept map requires the students to identify and organize information and to establish meaningful relationships between the pieces of information.
- Gaming: Gaming represents another method to engage learners, such as *Jeopardy!* or *Wheel of Fortune*. Games energize learners, who find it fun and exciting to participate and test their retention. Games also provide prompt feedback to the educator.
- Case Illustration: Ask students to think of a case to illustrate a principle presented or a future application of the material.
- Restate Key Points: Ask students to restate the material in their own words on a piece of paper.
- Stump Your Partner: Ask students to turn to their neighbor come up with a question that they feel is very difficult. Collect the questions verbally or on index cards for use in other lectures, in practice, or on exams.
- Note Check: Ask students to turn to their partner and compare notes, focusing on the most important points of the preceding content. What are they most confused about? Collect these comments either verbally or on index cards.
- Debates
- Brainstorming
- Role-plays
- Mock interviews

End/Conclusion

Summarize the major concepts succinctly at the end of the lecture or have students summarize the key points. Remind the learners what has been accomplished during the presentation, how it is relevant to them, and what they should do with this knowledge. This summary provides a chance to repeat and emphasize the major points, allows the lecturer and/or learners to tie up any loose ends, and provides a sense of closure for the audience. The lecturer can end with a provocative thought, summary of the major issue, quotation, or preview of coming material. It is useful to provide further resources. If the lecture is part of an ongoing course, provide a bridge to the next class by previewing readings, assignments, or key concepts to come. The summary also helps learners remember any questions they may have had during the lecture. Stay after class for a few minutes to answer any questions (See Table 6.1).

Table 6.1 Guidelines for an effective lecture

Tip	Principle
Preparation	
Know the context	Understand the purpose of the lecture
Know the audience	Anticipate learners' preexisting knowledge base and cognitive structure
	Determine what will be relevant, interesting to learner
	Understanding how the material may be applied in the future
Know the content	Include knowledge, skills, and attitudes
	Narrow scope of content to enhance learning and retention
Develop a logical organizational schema	Promotes ability to focus, follow, and understand
Introduction	
Attend to the learning climate	Promotes interest and participation
Pretest questions (*optional*)	Provides audience feedback and increases attention
State learning objectives	Establish lecture purpose, relevance and organization
Get learner attention: video clip? Case? Question? etc.	Gain interest of audience
	Establish relevance
Provide outline	Preview of lecture
	Establish organizational map
Refer to previous learning	Connect with preexisting knowledge of learner
	Increases retention

(continued)

Table 6.1 (continued)

Tip	Principle
Middle	
Limit content	Helps manage information
	Increases retention
Use examples, anecdotes, cases	Promotes interest
	Improves clarity and understanding
Utilize visual aids	Enhances retention
Reviews at end of each section	Repetition promotes retention
	Focuses
Interactive strategy	Offer opportunity for knowledge/skill application
	Provides feedback on how well learner and lecturer are doing
	Enhances retention
Provide handouts	Offer opportunity for application
	Encourages self-directed learning
Closing	
Post test questions (*optional*)	Feedback, appraising performance/providing feedback
	Adding questions for audience feedback
Summarize: Integrate new information with previous information	Integration
	Repetition
	Increases retention
	Re-establishes relevance and application
Stay for questions	Feedback to learner and lecturer
Evaluation	
Collect data on impact of lecture	Improve learning
Student option or achievement	Improve lecture
Peer or group feedback	
Self-assessment with or without video	

Audiovisual Aids

Audiovisual aids such as white or blackboards, flip charts, or electronic slides (e.g., PowerPoint) can increase learning clarity and interest and therefore improve understanding and learning. Visual displays also have been shown to facilitate retention [25]. Such aids can help explain or reinforce key points in a lecture and provide a stimulus for discussion. Given that the majority of adults are visual or visual-multimodal learners [26] and tend to prefer visuals to text [27], adding audiovisual aids can help the efficacy of the overall presentation.

Audiovisual aids should be simple, clear, and uncluttered. No matter which aid you use, make sure that you talk to the audience and not the board, slides, or computer screen. If using a chalkboard or whiteboard, make sure to write with large, legible letters and ensure that those in the back can hear and/or see what you are presenting. Use multiple colors to emphasize points or draw diagrams. The most common audiovisual aid now is an electronic slideshow. Check the equipment for good functioning before starting the lecture. The actual audiovisual device chosen is less important than the appropriate use of it.

Stahl and Davis [28] provide key tips regarding the development of an electronic slideshow, including the following:

- Emphasize "data ink," or the substantive parts of data that change (dots, lines, labels, etc.), over "non-data ink," which represents the vehicle in which substantive data are presented (e.g., title, scales). This can be done skillfully utilizing PowerPoint "builds," for example, where by keeping the "non-data ink" constant, each successive slide depicts only the critical data that change, allowing the learners' attention to focus on the changes [29].
- Present data in "small multiples" [29] or groups of information at a time. As each "small multiple" is added, learners' attention is directed toward contrasting the differences and similarities to the former bit of information. The use of "small multiples" also allows the speaker to modulate the pace of learning.
- Transmit new knowledge both orally and visually. Learners tend to process visual and auditory input simultaneously. However, the sources must be synchronized and mutually reinforced to enhance learning [30].
- Use visuals with simultaneous oral narratives rather than visuals with text. The former has been shown to impact learning positively. Eliminate redundant text and avoid presenting orally a slightly different text than what is noted on the slide, which will distract learners.

- Present text and images in close proximity rather than far from each other on a slide [30]. Presenting words and pictures simultaneously versus successively also enhances learning.
- Eliminate legends and put labels directly on data to prevent breaking up the spatial contiguity of slides. Identify key points on each slide and eliminate excess information.
- Present bullet points in parallel structure, starting each with the same type of word (verb, noun, etc.). As a result, the learner's eye will tend to focus on the new information in each bullet.
- When presenting complicated images or diagrams, superimpose them on each other sequentially to emphasize what is changing and the associated similarities and differences of the data.
- "Builds" can be a powerful technique to present data but take time to develop. To be effective, the lecturer should anticipate each slide with the audience before showing it. Therefore, the lecturer must be familiar with the slides and would do well to rehearse the presentation rather than relying on the slides as lecture notes.

Direct the learners' attention to the key features. Make sure to give adequate time for the audience to review and possibly copy the information. There is no need to talk during this time. Beware not to use audiovisual aids excessively. If you are using video or audio technology, make sure that students know what to watch for during the presentation. Make sure to provide ample time for discussion and summary of the relevant points.

Performance Behaviors

The teacher's behavior during a lecture can significantly affect the efficacy of the presentation. Nonverbal lecture behaviors have a substantial effect on speaker credibility and persuasiveness [31]. Consider speech patterns, voice quality, vocabulary, mannerisms, facial expressions, appearance, posture, and eye contact, all of which can add to the persuasiveness and interest of a presentation [31].

Prepare yourself emotionally. Some lecturers listen to music before speaking; others spend time reviewing their notes; still others might walk through the empty classroom, gathering their thoughts. Determine what activity might promote energy and focus for you to present with confidence and enthusiasm [32].

Rehearse. Rehearse your presentation to ensure that it fits within the allotted time frame. Though time consuming, rehearsing is particularly helpful for an inexperienced instructor. Rehearsal can lead to improvement of fluency, decreased reliance on reading slides or notes, and decreased fidgeting and nervousness.

Arrive in class early. Use your voice informally with the students before you begin the lecture so that your tone can maintain its conversational quality [33]. Take a few deep breaths or tighten and release all the muscles in your whole body to promote relaxation and minimize nervousness. Once you get started, anxiety will fade [33].

Establish rapport with students. By creating a warm, personal, direct, and conversational relationship with the audience from the outset, the lecturer will help students feel more engaged in the class. This engagement also gives students a sense that the lecturer is speaking to each one individually. Eye contact can increase learning partly by acting as an arousal stimulus to the learner and, therefore, facilitate the encoding of information. Gaze-aversion may have the opposite effect [34]. Throughout the lecture, maintain eye contact with individual students one at a time. Avoid aimless scanning of the audience. Try not to lock on to one student—a glance lasting more than 5 s will make a student uncomfortable. Some lecturers divide the lecture hall into sections and address comments and questions and direct eye contact to each section during the course of a lecture. If direct eye contact affects your concentration, look between two students or at foreheads. Concentrate on the attentive learners but do not avoid the non-listeners. By focusing on the students as if speaking to a small group, you will not only increase their attentiveness but also be able to notice their facial expressions and body movements. Such responses will help inform you as to whether you are speaking too slowly or too fast and give you feedback as to whether the students understand the material [33].

Avoid reading your lecture notes. Reading interferes with maintaining eye contact with your audience and leads to a distancing experience. Use note cards or slides as guides only. Make sure that they are easily visible so that a quick glance is all you need.

Be Enthusiastic. Enthusiasm is highly correlated with overall teaching effectiveness in student ratings of teachers [35]. Convey enthusiasm for students through looking at them, using their names, and inviting them to ask questions. Humor, energy, and passion can also convey enthusiasm. These behaviors motivate learning, spark interest in the topic, and maintain interest in the lecture.

Strive for natural conversation. Attempt to create a natural, spontaneous conversation with your students or the audience as a whole. Vary your pitch, and use inflections and tones as if in natural conversation. A more expressive delivery will result from focusing on the meaning of what you are saying.

Vary speech patterns. Vocal variety and verbal pauses can provide energy, boost interest, and provide excitement to a lecture. Project your voice so that it can be heard easily at the back of the room. Pauses can be used for emphasis, a transition from one idea to the next, or after a rhetorical question. Slower speech allows learners to comprehend information more easily, as well as take notes. It also can be used to emphasize important topics. However, if the lecturer speaks too slowly, students may become bored.

Language. Utilize simple, clear, and dramatic language. Avoid vague terms (e.g., "sometimes," "often"), jargon, or empty words.

Body Movement. Look professional and relaxed. Occasionally move about the room. Physical movement can increase interest, emphasize key ideas, communicate feelings, and create connection with an audience. By moving around, the instructor can show his or her face to the largest number of audience members, which is an effective communication technique. Movement also can convey that an instructor is comfortable with a presentation. Use purposeful, sustained gestures as well as an open, casual stance to invite students' questions. Avoid aimless, stereotypical movements or gestures, which can be distracting (e.g., shuffling notes, fidgeting).

Keep track of time. If you are running out of time, avoid speeding up to cover all your material. Plan in advance what parts you can leave out, should it be necessary. Have handouts of material ready if there is not enough time to cover the content verbally. Some lecturers prepare their presentation in 10-min segments so that if they run over due to learner questions or a need to clarify particular areas more carefully, the lecturer can easily drop out a section of the previously planned talk without affecting the general flow of material. The section should usually come from the middle of the talk, because the lecturer would not want to short-change the ending.

Manage the nerves. Strategies to cope with nervousness include good preparation, mastery of the material, knowing your audience, and rehearsing for success.

Evaluation

The final component of providing an effective lecture is the evaluation, which provides feedback so that learners can see if they are accurately integrating the new material while allowing the instructor to discover whether or not he or she presented the material in a clear and understandable manner. Therefore, the goal is twofold—to improve learning and to aid one's ability to lecture. Student opinion, student achievement, peer feedback, and reflection on practice represent the different types of evaluations and are discussed in the subsequent text.

Student opinions: Obtaining student assessments of the teaching can be achieved through informal conversation with students or through an evaluation form. Focus groups, rating scales, or written reports can also be used. The difficulty with focus groups is that they are time consuming and can be hijacked by an outspoken participant. Rating schedules often tell a lecturer what is good or bad but rarely how to improve a lecture. Written reports can also be time consuming. The lecturer could invite comments about the lecture via an electronic discussion board, if available, where students could identify topics they did not understand, ask questions, or give feedback on the presentation.

Other approaches include having students fill out a brief, three-item evaluation (i.e., "what was useful, what was not useful, and suggestions for improvement") after *each* lecture or write a "minute paper" where students are asked to respond in one or two sentences to the following questions: (1) What stood out as most important in today's lecture? (2) What are you confused about? Both methods provide time for the learner to reflect on the new material while also providing the lecturer feedback on his or her teaching skills through critiques of the teaching techniques and information on how learning occurred.

Student Achievement: Testing can also suggest the success of a given lecture—particularly if done immediately following the lecture. If testing is done at the end of a learning sequence, the results might better reflect the student's capacity to master the material through outside reading or studying of lecture notes instead of demonstrating understanding or retention gained primarily from a given lecture.

Peer Feedback: Though time consuming, peer feedback is an important adjunct to student evaluations. This feedback can be set up as a mutual evaluation, where one lecturer observes another and vice versa, each providing feedback to the other through the use of a rating schedule [36], checklist [37], or discussion. Such feedback can serve to encourage effective behaviors and diminish or eliminate ineffective ones.

Reflective Practice: Using a reflective approach has become a key part of continuing professional development [38, 39]. The approach involves several strategies:

- Collect and analyze any student or peer evaluations.
- Make notes to yourself after each lecture—consider the timing, effectiveness, and appropriateness of examples. Did you feel your explanations were clear? Did your audience appear engaged? Was the amount of material covered appropriate given the abilities, experience, and motivation of the students? Were the visual aids clear and of the right length?
- Make note of any comments or questions asked by students. Did students seem to obtain what you intended from the activities? Did the material provided complement the lecture?
- Evaluate how well you met students' learning objectives.

On the basis of these findings, adjust the lecture. Sharing individual reflections on practice with members of a group or course team can facilitate improving the overall quality of lecturers in the department or faculty.

Observing yourself via video or audio is another very effective technique to use in improving the quality of your presentation skills. Periodically record your lectures. Is your tone conversational? Did you provide clear transitions? Did you use effective pauses or emphasize the material in other ways? Did you clearly respond to questions and maintain good eye contact? How did the learning climate feel? Whether done by yourself or with a mentor or a peer evaluator, identify both desirable and undesirable behaviors, and then set goals for improving the quality. A lecture skills checklist can also be used.

Words to the Wise
- Invest time preparing! Carefully consider your audience and the context in which you are asked to present a lecture before determining exactly what content you will present. Select the best organizational schema and develop a logical presentation.
- Develop clear learner objectives. Make the objectives relevant, realistic, observable, measurable, learner focused, and clearly stated. Do they involve more than one of the key educational domains—knowledge, skills, and attitudes?
- Less is more! Do not overload your lecture with facts and details. Limit the key concepts and back them up with clear examples and other strategies to enhance clarity.
- Foster active learning. Provide time for learners to apply their new knowledge and receive feedback.
- Reflect on your lecture performance. Ask for feedback from students and peers and self-assess. What kinds of questions did learners ask? Did learners appear or act engaged? What seemed to puzzle your learners?

Ask Your Mentor or Colleagues
- Are there teaching workshops in our institution to help educate me about being an effective teacher?
- Could you or another expert teacher observe a lecture with or without the use of videotape and provide concrete feedback?
- What have you found to be the most significant lessons learned from giving a lecture? What pitfalls should I look out for with regard to lecturing?
- What have you found to be the most effective form of lecturing?
- What do you do if the audience resists engagement?

References

1. General Medical Council. Tomorrow's doctors. Recommendations on undergraduate medical education, vol. 2. London, UK: General Medical Council; 2003.
2. Costa ML, van Rensburg L, Rushton N. Does teaching style matter? A randomized trial of group discussion versus lecturers in orthopaedic undergraduate teaching. Med Educ. 2007;41:214–7.
3. Association of American Medical Colleges. CurrMIT (Curriculum Management & Information Tool). 2011. https://www.aamc.org/initiatives/medaps/curriculumreports/264656/topicteachingandassessmentformats.html . Accessed 1 Dec 2011.
4. Clark JM, Houston TK, Kolodner K, Branch WT, Levine RB, Kern DE. Teaching the teachers. National survey of faculty development in departments of medicine of US teaching hospitals. J Gen Intern Med. 2004;19:205–14.
5. Arredondo MA, Busch E, Douglass HO, Petrelli NJ. The use of video-taped lectures in surgical oncology. J Cancer Educ. 1994;9(2):86–9.
6. Bligh DA. What's the use of lectures? San Francisco, CA: Jossey-Bass; 2000.
7. Cardall S, Krupat E, Ulrich M. Live lecture versus video-recorded lecture: are students voting with their feet? Acad Med. 2008;83(12):1174–8.
8. Fyrenius A, Bergdahl B, Silen C. Med Teach. 2005;27(1):61–5.
9. Knowles MS. The adult learner: a neglected species. 3rd ed. Houston, TX: Gulf; 1984.

10. Brown G, Manogue M. AMEE Medical Education Guide No 22. Refreshing lecturing: a guide for lecturers. Med Teach. 2001;23:231–44.
11. Miller GA. The magical number seven, plus or minus two: some limits to our capacity for processing information. Psychol Rev. 1956;63:81–97.
12. Christenson CM. Relationships between pupil achievement, pupil affect-need, teacher warmth, and teacher permissiveness. J Educ Psychol. 1960;51(3):169–74.
13. Ausubel D. Alternative theories of retention and forgetting. Educational psychology: a cognitive view. New York: Holt, Rinehart and Winston; 1968.
14. Ernst H, Colthorpe K. The efficiency of interactive lecturing for students with diverse science backgrounds. Adv Physiol Educ. 2007;31:41–4.
15. Mayer R. Learning and instruction. New Jersey: Pearson Education; 2003.
16. Brown GA, Armstrong S. On explaining. In: Wragg EC, editor. Classroom teaching skills. London, UK: Croom Helm; 1983.
17. Gibbs G, Jenkins A. Break up your lectures: or Christaller sliced up. J Geogr Higher Educ. 1984;8(1):27–39.
18. Ebert-May D, Brewer C, Allred S. Innovation in large lectures—Teaching for active learning. Bioscience. 1997;47(9):601–7.
19. Homme J, Grath A, Morgenstern B. Utilization of an audience response system. Med Educ. 2004;38:55–9.
20. Uhari M, Renko M, Soin H. Experiences of using an interactive audience response system in lectures. BMC Med Educ. 2003;3:12.
21. Pradhan A, Sparano D, Ananth C. The influence of an audience response system on knowledge retention: an application to resident education. Am J Obstet Gynecol. 2005;193:1827–30.
22. Kaleta R, Joosten T. Student response system: a University of Wisconsin system study of clickers. Educause Center for Applied Research Bulletin. 8 May 2007;10:1–12.
23. Tomorrow's professor. Improving the effectiveness of your lectures. MSG #495 guided notes. 2007. http://ctl.stanford.edu/TompProf/postings/495.html . Accessed 15 Nov 2011.
24. Public speaking tips. Creating quality handouts. 29 Dec 2003. www.speaking-tips.com/articles/creating-quality-handouts.aspx. Accessed 14 Dec 2011.
25. Levie WH, Lentz R. Effects of text illustrations: a review of research. Educ Commun Technol J. 1982;30(4):195–232.
26. Baycan Z, Nacar M. Learning styles of first year medical students attending Erciyes University in Kayseri, Turkey. Adv Physiol Educ. 2007;31(2):158–60.
27. Price L. Lecturers' vs. students' perceptions of the accessibility of instructional materials. Instr Sci. 2007;35(4):317–41.
28. Stahl SM, Davis RL. Best practices for medical educators. Carlsbad, CA: NEI; 2009.
29. Tufte E. The visual display of quantitative information. 2nd ed. Cheshire, CT: Graphics; 1983.

30. Mayer R, Moreno R. Nine ways to reduce cognitive load in multimedia learning. Educ Psychologist 2003;38(1):43–52.
31. Burgoon JK, Birk T, Pfau M. Nonverbal behaviors, persuasion, and credibility. Hum Commun Res. 1990;17:140–69.
32. Lowman J. Mastering the techniques of teaching. San Francisco, CA: Jossey-Bass; 1984.
33. Davis B. Delivering a Lecture. In: Davis B. Tools for teaching. San Francisco, CA: Jossey-Bass; 1993.
34. Fullwood C, Doherty-Sneddon G. Effect of gazing at the camera during a video link on recall. Appl Ergon. 2006;37(2):167–75.
35. Irby DM. Clinical teacher effectiveness in medicine. J Med Educ. 1978;53:808–15.
36. Newman LR, Lown BA, Jones RN, Johansson A, Schwartzstein RM. Developing a peer assessment of lecturing instrument: lessons learned. Acad Med. 2009;84:1104–10.
37. Sullivan RL, McIntosh N. Delivering effective lectures. JHPIEGO strategy paper #5. US Agency for International Development. Dec 1996. www.jhpiego.jhu.edu . Accessed 15 Oct 2011.
38. Brooksfeld S. Becoming a critically reflective teacher. San Francisco, CA: Jossey-Bass; 1995.
39. Schon D. Educating the reflective practitioner. San Francisco, CA: Jossey-Bass; 1987.

How to Use Technology in Educational Innovation

7

John Luo, Robert Boland, and Carlyle H. Chan

In years past, faculty in an academic medical center taught primarily either in the clinical setting via supervision or in a classroom setting in the form of a lecture. Teaching was in "real time" with direct interaction and immediate questions and answers during this time period. Faculty often spoke at length from their notes, and students scrambled to write down the many "pearls" of wisdom. Overhead projectors and large bulletin boards were the medium where teachers often illustrated a lesson or provided a summary outline of the information covered. Many faculty members remember the "analog" days with fondness because mastery of the material was the focus, not the teaching methodology. Learning how to use an overhead projector was easy since it was as intuitive as using a pen.

The Internet and new computer technologies have dramatically changed the teaching methodology for faculty today. Presentation software such as Microsoft PowerPoint and Apple Keynote provide greater visual stimulation during educational sessions with multimedia video, animations, and graphs to capture or focus the

J. Luo, M.D. (✉)
Department of Psychiatry, UCLA Semel Institute for Neuroscience and Human Behavior, 760 Westwood Plaza, Los Angeles, CA, USA
e-mail: jsluo@mednet.ucla.edu

© Springer International Publishing Switzerland 2016
L.W. Roberts (ed.), *The Clinician Educator Guidebook*,
DOI 10.1007/978-3-319-27980-0_7

attention of the audience. LCD projectors with a laptop computer are "de rigueur" for lecture delivery in every setting imaginable. The Internet over the last 15 years has evolved from a collection of interconnected static Web pages into a rich repository of educational content with a dizzying array of options such as audio, video, databases, and much more.

Today, faculty with their increasing time demands for research, clinical care, and administration need to find innovative ways to impart their knowledge and incorporate their teaching skills. Educators need to expand their repertoire with new teaching technologies or risk being perceived as limited and ineffective Luddites. Fortunately, the learning curve for many of these new technologies has diminished and a second degree in computer programming is no longer necessary. Web-based educational methods have become one of the more popular areas of focus with its broad reach across large distances and availability 24/7.

Traditional educators are saddened with the decreased emphasis on direct teaching methods, and may even doubt the effectiveness of Web-based educational materials. Maloney et al. compared Web-based versus face-to-face fall prevention short courses for health professionals in a randomized controlled trial [1]. They determined that face-to-face and Web-based delivery modalities produced comparable outcomes for participation, satisfaction, knowledge acquisition, and change in practice. In addition, their study demonstrated more cost-effectiveness in the break-even analysis for Web-based education. The barriers to learning how to create these Web-based materials have all but dissipated, as software tools have become easier to learn and educators have become much more tech savvy. In this chapter, we review examples of Web-based educational methods and provide cases of their use.

Web-Based Educational Methods

Engaging in Web-based education can assume four different roles: accessing information, creation of educational content, collaboration, and management of educational content.

Access

Accessing involves learning about the various Web-based resources available to supplement and enhance educational objectives. The single largest compendium of medical education materials is the AAMC site, www.MedEdPortal.com. This site contains peer-reviewed teaching resources, assessment tools, and faculty development materials. It is organized by topic and by specialty, and worth reviewing for inspiration. Faculty members who have developed their own online creations may submit them to the MedEdPortal, which once accepted counts as a refereed multimedia publication on a curriculum vitae (CV).

The LIFE Curriculum (Learning to address Impairment and Fatigue to Enhance patient safety) (www.lifecurriculum.info) produced by Duke University Hospital in conjunction with UNC Hospitals, the NC AHEC, and the NC Physician's Health Program provides materials to address fatigue and stress. This curriculum utilizes videos from MedicalCrossfire.com, a continuing medical education Web site, as well as videos created by the site authors to demonstrate scenarios of discussions heard in a residents lounge that trigger teaching points. The teaching guides and self-assessment tools are great examples of materials that support Web-based learning.

In addition to its entertainment value, www.youtube.com has become a resource for instructional videos. Individuals and companies have posted tutorials on various topics and products. For example, medical school faculty members have uploaded teaching demonstrations. Patients describe their signs, symptoms, and clinical course. All of this rich material is free for viewing, including any copyrighted materials, since the copyright owners often elect to leave a snippet of their materials on YouTube in order to market to their fans, gain market insight, and generate ad revenue.

Content Development

Presentation software such as PowerPoint and Keynote (for Mac) are popular tools used to create online education materials. Educators tend to create linear lectures that can be overcrowded with information. *Presentation Zen* (www.presentationzen.com) is a blog and book that offers strategies to produce more readable slides, such as limiting the text to show only visuals, not what you intend to say [2]. More educators now embed videos into their presentations, which leads to common mistakes during the creation of online presentations. Typically, the location of the video is linked to the slide when the author actually intended to include the video. A quick tip to determine if the video was properly inserted is to look at the presentation file size, which should reflect the addition of the video file size. An alternative to the presentations generated by PowerPoint and Keynote is to use Prezi (www.prezi.com). It utilizes more movement and less linear sequencing, which creates a dynamic presentation using constructivist learning theory which is more focused on the relationship of concepts and building a deeper understanding of a topic than plain static content.

Developing content for distribution via the Internet once entailed mastering complicated video presentation/editing software. Now, at the touch of a button, PowerPoint add-on software such as Camtasia (www.techsmith.com/camtasia.html) or video screen capture software such as Camstudio (www.camstudio.org) records the audio portion of a presentation and synchronizes it with the slides being shown. This process easily creates a "webcast" of a traditional lecture with a live audience or a specific lecture intended for Web-based learning.

Once the video presentation has been recorded, it may be distributed as a "podcast" in addition to being available on a Web site. A "podcast" is a term coined by Apple Inc. for the process of adding an RSS (resource distribution framework site summary, a.k.a. really simple syndication) document to the audio or video file. This RSS file is basically XML code known also as a "feed." It is used to make Web site content available, such as a video presentation, to multiple other Web sites or specific "feed reader" software, which keeps track of new and updated content. The RSS code also enables educators to deliver podcasts directly from their university Web site for downloading. Educational podcasts can also be distributed via Apple's iTunes University, which a number of faculty at many well-known universities have done.

Adobe Authorware (www.adobe.com/products/authorware/) is a more sophisticated program used to create multimedia online educational materials and DVDs. It has features such as polls and quizzes that help emphasize certain key learning points, as well as a timeline to facilitate development of learning progress. Adobe is no longer developing new versions of Authorware, but continues to sell this product. Articulate (www.articulate.com) is another e-learning package to consider for its additional tools beyond PowerPoint and podcasts. Regardless of the software used to create content, the next step is to ensure that it is Advanced Distributed Learning Shareable Courseware Object Reference Model (ADL SCORM) compliant. The ADL Initiative was established in 1997 by the Department of Defense to standardize and modernize training and education management and delivery. Compliance or conformance with SCORM ensures that the product can be moved across various learning management system (LMS) platforms. Google offers a SCORM Compliance Test to view the product in various ways, and then determine SCORM status.

Most simulations are geared towards mimicking the interactions typical of a psychiatric encounter, and therefore need a high level of sophistication and quality that are challenging to produce. Some straightforward techniques such as medication treatment decisions, evaluation of serious side effects, or rehearsal for management of rare critical events lend themselves to computer modeling [3]. In the absence of this level of artificial intelligence, some educators have constructed innovative uses of virtual spaces as educational tools. For example, Dr. Daniel Freedman created a virtual neutral space to gauge participant reactions [4]. Yellowlees and colleagues [5] made use of the virtual community Second Life to create an environment meant to mimic what it feels like to be psychotic—in this space the learner walks through a building where pictures change from neutral to threatening themes and a bodiless voice urges them to kill themselves. Students using this simulation felt that it helped them to understand what it must be like to be paranoid. Simulation technologies are poised to be a major area of innovation in the future: with advances in artificial intelligence as well as contributions from the field of computer gaming industry, one can anticipate simulations that approach realistic human interactions.

Collaboration

Collaborating with colleagues from different academic institutions has become easier with the Internet. When coauthoring a paper, book chapter, or presentation, these documents can be shared in the "cloud." Cloud computing is where both the software program and the data are stored and delivered from the Internet server. The only requirement of the desktop or laptop computer is to have a Web browser. Google Docs (www.docs.google.com) allows access and editing of a file from any location with an Internet-connected computing device, including tablets and smartphones. Many educators have used Microsoft Word's "track changes" option to highlight each contributor's additions or corrections in a different color and with strike outs along with the option to accept or reject the changes; however the static nature of Word requires the changes to be made one person at a time. Cloud-based services have a similar feature to compare across multiple drafts as well as track different file versions, and authors can simultaneously contribute to the document. DropBox (www.dropbox.com) is another popular cloud-based service because it provides a shared space online and on the computer where multiple users can easily update one another with their contributions without sending them as attachments via e-mail. Once the software service is installed, the local computer DropBox folder is automatically synchronized to the cloud when the computer is connected online. Collaborators can share specific folders in their DropBox account so that everyone gets an updated copy of whatever is put in the shared folder.

The Web 2.0 online environment offers other methods of asynchronous collaboration. For example, a wiki allows multiple authors to collaborate in creating an online document: the potential of this method is exemplified by the popular Wikipedia. This online encyclopedia has become one of the most popular online reference sources in the world and has the advantage over traditional resources of being continuously updated. Although the accuracy of the information included is dependent on the expertise of the writer, the theory behind the wiki is that in an open environment where every participant is an editor, any errors will be discovered and improved. This process is borne out by the fact that

Wikipedia compares favorably to traditional general reference resources with traditional editing [6]. However, the success of this wiki is the result of the many thousands of contributors to the document and the enormous collective time spent on both content creation and editing [7]. Most educators who desire to create a wiki find that the smaller critical mass of interested editors at their disposal makes wiki creation more of a challenge.

Nonetheless, wiki can be useful in education. It is tempting to imagine the creation of an online textbook of psychiatry that would obviate the need for expensive resources. Sadly, the academic system is not conducive to the amount of work and time that would be required for such a project. The anonymity, lack of copyright protection, and lack of peer review are emblematic of the wiki tradition but are an anathema to the academic process. Despite these limitations, there are practical uses for a wiki within a training program. For example, some residencies have used a wiki structure to create and maintain a "resident's handbook" or "studying pearls." The ease of access and ability to constantly update the document make it ideal for this purpose [8]. Many educational institutions maintain wiki platforms at their institutional Web site that are free for their faculty and residents to use. Educators without these resources can utilize free online wiki services. The reference site Wikimatrix (www.wikimatrix.com) maintains a list of available wiki sites and software, and it has detailed feature comparisons.

Online conferencing can allow a team to meet virtually. This approach is useful for situations in which the learning team is geographically remote. In such cases, online conferencing services (such as Skype™ and GoToMeeting™) are available at no or low cost. Virtual tele- or videoconferencing can have a variety of formats. In education, the most common method is the "one-to-many" conferencing format in which the teacher uses the technology to, in essence, lecture to a large crowd. The setup for this generally includes a screen for presenting slides and other visual content, including, potentially, a visual of the speaker. The advantage is one of practicality—an educator can efficiently disseminate information to a large group who may be at various locations. In these settings, information is primarily transmitted in one direction in that the lecturer spends most of the time transmitting the video and audio to a large audience, who are most often muted for the majority of the session. Given the general lack of interactivity, one may question the value of this format at all versus, for example, a recorded lecture that can be sent to the students. Therefore, before planning such a conference one should consider whether a prerecorded option would better serve the purpose. Videoconference lectures should be considered when some interactivity is preferred. In these cases the interactivity must be well organized. Most often spontaneous audio questioning is not possible in larger groups; questions are preferably submitted through a text-based chat option and most videoconferencing software allows for this chat function to be used simultaneous to the presentation. During the presentation, the lecturer can view online questions submitted by the crowd which can be either taken as a group at the end of the presentation or handled during various points in the presentation. The advantage of the latter approach is that the audience feedback can be used to guide the presentation, and, in part, compensate for the lack of visual feedback that typically helps a live lecturer know whether the audience is being engaged at the right level.

Although this method can be useful for traditional lecture-style teaching, modern medical education is moving away from tradition lecture styles to interactive formats in which trainees are responsible for the learning process and teachers serve more as facilitators. An example is team-based learning (TBL), which requires greater interactivity. Although most TBL groups prefer face-to-face learning, in situations where this is impractical (e.g., residents are at different facilities) videoconferencing offers a viable solution. Using videoconferencing for the type of group discussion typical of TBL requires some training (for example, to compensate for the decrease in nonverbal cues); however, with practice and proper facilitation most groups can adapt successfully, and a number of training programs have successfully used this technology [9]. One cannot emphasize too greatly the importance of understanding how virtual interactions differ from real ones. Participants tend to see online interactions as more formal and less spontaneous than face-to-face interactions, and the facilitator of an online meeting must work hard to assure that all participants have a chance to participate.

Although this type of videoconferencing solves the problem of distance, it still requires the participants to be available for a real-time discussion. Such meetings can be a challenge for trainees who may have varied schedules and responsibilities. It is therefore tempting to consider the option of using asynchronous communication to facilitate TBL. Opinions vary regarding whether real-time interactions are crucial to the process of TBL. Some groups are experimenting with asynchronous team learning using bulletin board style postings entered at the team member's convenience [10].

Content Management

Managing educational content is made easier by the use of Course Management Systems (CMS), also known as an LMS or Virtual Learning Environment (VLE) software systems. e-Learning software has the advantage of being asynchronous, i.e., available 24 h, 7 days a week and available via Internet connection. The software can be used for a stand-alone teaching module or as a distance learning course or it can be used to facilitate or augment a live course. Typically, such software permits the posting of a course syllabus with hypertext linkages to other Web sources, viewing of uploaded videos, slide presentations, portable document format (PDF) readings, quizzes, chat rooms, bulletin board threads, grade books, etc. Chat rooms permit an instructor to conduct live virtual office hours while bulletin boards facilitate asynchronous discussions.

There are many proprietary products such as BlackBoard (www.blackboard.com), whose pricing varies depending on the number of sites, users, etc. Sakai (www.sakaiproject.org), Joomla (www.joomla.org), and Moodle (www.moodle.org) are open-source versions (source code is freely available to use). Proprietary systems can be costly but open-source systems require Information Technology department support to implement unless the educator has sufficient technology savvy and access to the Web site server. A more extensive listing of current LMS may be found at www.softwareshortlist.com/software/learning_management_system_LMS_directory.

The existence of e-Learning does not obviate the need for sound educational pedagogy. In fact, it may require stricter attention to content development. The ADDIE model of instructional design is frequently used. This entails the stages of *analysis* (defining *what* is to be learned), *design* (specifying *how* it is to be learned), *development* (authoring and creating the program), *implementation* (going "live"), and *evaluation* (assessing the success or failure of learning. While sequential, there are ongoing feedback loops to shape each stage. Embedded in the ADDIE stages are other pedagogy issues such as Bloom's hierarchical taxonomy of educational objectives, Edgar Dale's Cone of Learning, and Kirkpatrick's four levels of organizing program evaluation [11].

HIPAA, Fair Use, and Creative Commons Copyright

Creating digital media for the Internet means that content can easily be reproduced, both legally and illegally, and then disseminated across the World Wide Web. There are several implications of this ability. First, patient-identifiable content should be avoided. Even with HIPAA-compliant signed video releases for educational purposes, patient images can reach unintended audiences. Also, once an object reaches the Internet, it never really disappears as it may be captured and preserved on some obscure or remote server. Using actors with signed contractual releases to simulate clinical situations obviates this concern.

Secondly, anything published is under copyright, even without the circled c logo "©." Fair use implies the limited reproduction of copyrighted materials without fee under certain circumstances. Using, for example, a published illustration once to illustrate a point to a group of residence might be permissible, but placing that illustration on a Web site without authorization would not. Fair use rules are explained in more detail at school library Web sites.

Finally, creative commons copyright is a vehicle to freely license materials. CC copyright meets that an author agrees that others are free to use the author's creations as long as they attribute the author. There are some further restrictions one may stipulate if desired, e.g., others may not change an author's creation without authorization, or a creation may not be used for commercial purposes. There are actually six license variations and the details may be reviewed at www.creativecommons.org.

Conclusion

The advantages of Web-based education are tremendous, well beyond mere multimedia use and distance learning. Web-based educational content is easily created with PowerPoint presentations using the save-to-Web feature. Lectures can be captured to be broadcast later online via podcasts. More sophisticated educational modules with video, tables, graphs, and quizzes can be created with LMS. Collaboration or TBL can occur in real time or in an asynchronous nature with the use of LMS, cloud-based computing, wikis, or videoconferencing. It used to be that Web-based materials required sufficient technology savvy, including programming skills and knowledge of client–server technology. Nowadays, many of these tools demand less technical skill but more appropriate instructional design to educate the learner with the right methodology. The time, effort, and creativity to develop these Web-based educational materials are no longer just a labor of love, but now recognized as an academic activity worthy to be listed in one's curriculum vitae.

Words to the Wise
- Do not be afraid to transform your teaching material into a new way of learning.
- Start with products available at your institution, such as an LMS.
- There are no mistakes, only learning opportunities, with technology.
- Analyze, design, develop, implement, and evaluate. Repeat.

Ask Your Mentor or Colleagues
- What inspired you to use that software or technology?
- How much time did it take to learn to use it?
- If you had to do it over again, would you use the same software or something else?
- How much technical support did your institution provide?

References

1. Maloney S, Haas R, Keating JL, Molloy E, Jolly B, Sims J, Morgan P, Haines T. Breakeven, cost benefit, cost effectiveness, and willingness to pay for web-based versus face-to-face education delivery for health professionals. J Med Internet Res. 2012;14(2):e47.
2. Reynolds G. Presentation zen. Berkeley, CA: New Riders; 2008.
3. Benjamin S, Margariti M. Technology for psychiatric educators. In: Gask L, Coskun B, Baron D, editors. Teaching psychiatry: putting theory into practice. London: Wiley; 2011.
4. Freeman D, Pugh K, Antley A, Slater M, Bebbington P, Gittins M, Dunn G, Kuipers E, Fowler D, Garety P. Virtual reality study of paranoid thinking in the general population. Br J Psychiatry. 2008;192(4):258–63. http://www.youtube.com/watch?v=rUF_7HGYWiI.
5. Yellowlees PM, Cook JN. Education about hallucinations using an internet virtual reality system: a qualitative survey. Acad Psychiatry. 2006;30(6): 534–9.
6. Giles J. Internet encyclopaedias go head to head. Nature. 2005; 438(7070):900–1.
7. Thompson CL, Schulz WL, Terrence A. A student authored online medical education textbook: editing patterns and content evaluation of a medical student wiki. AMIA Annu Symp Proc. 2011;2011:1392–401. Epub 24 Dec 2011.
8. Chauhan M. Teaching with Technology. Presented at the 2009 Annual Meeting of the American Association of Directors of Residency Training. Available at: http://www.aadprt.org/pages.aspx?PanelID=0&PageName=Teaching_With_Technology.
9. Mash B, Marais D, Van Der Walt S, Van Deventer I, Steyn M, Labadarios D. Assessment of the quality of interaction in distance learning programmes utilizing the Internet or interactive television: perceptions of students and lecturers. Med Teach. 2006;28(1):e1–9. Epub 22 Apr 2006.
10. Morrison F, Zimmerman J, Hall M, Chase H, Kaushal R, Ancker JS. Developing an online and in-person HIT workforce training program using a team-based learning approach. AMIA Annu Symp Proc. 2011;2011:63–71.
11. Chan CH, Robbins LI. E-Learning systems: promises and pitfalls. Acad Psychiatry. 2006;30(6):491–7.

How to Approach Clinical Supervision

8

Michael D. Jibson, Michael I. Casher, and Sara R. Figueroa

听而易忘, ⊠ 而易, 做而易懂. --中国⊠⊠
I hear and I forget. I see and I remember.
I do and I understand.

Chinese proverb

Clinical supervision is the "parenting" of academic life. In no other setting are faculty attitudes so thoroughly modeled, responsibility for the trainee's work so totally assumed, control over real-time decisions so completely surrendered, knowledge of what trainees actually do so rarely verified, or preparatory training so wholly inadequate to the task. Happily, few faculty think through the full implications of the supervisory role before conceiving an academic career; otherwise, there might be no rising generation.

Also in common with parenting, however, are the satisfactions of supervision. No other setting offers faculty the potential for such impact on the quality of a trainee's practice for years beyond residency, engenders such depth and quality of relationships with nascent colleagues, or provides such wealth of opportunity for

M.D. Jibson, M.D., Ph.D. (⊠)
Department of Psychiatry, University of Michigan Health System,
1500 E. Medical Center Dr, Ann Arbor, MI, USA
e-mail: mdjibson@med.umich.edu

© Springer International Publishing Switzerland 2016
L.W. Roberts (ed.), *The Clinician Educator Guidebook*,
DOI 10.1007/978-3-319-27980-0_8

self-reflection and professional growth. After years of faculty service, few honors compare with the implicit accolade of the phrase, "I was trained by …."

The academic physician's assignment as a supervisor of trainees is an honor and a privilege that has been years in coming. Yet he or she may not have had—probably have not had—formal preparation for teaching in the clinical setting but likely learned through personal experiences as the recipient of supervision, through identification with respected teachers from his or her training. It is nonetheless important for the academic physician to formally review the role and reflect on the qualities he or she found most helpful (and otherwise) and those he or she most wants to emulate.

This chapter addresses both theoretical and practical aspects of clinical supervision. It is broadly divided into inpatient and outpatient settings, which differ in such fundamental qualities as depth of experience of the trainees, duration of oversight, and frequency of contact. Even so, all supervision has much in common, and lessons outlined in one section may be more broadly applied than this division implies.

The Psychology of the Attending/Trainee Relationship

Much has been written in the medical education literature about the best practices for optimal learning, and general medical education principles apply directly to hospital-based teaching and outpatient supervision. From a different perspective, the writings of the noted psychologist Erik Erikson have great relevance for the role of a supervisor in the lives of medical students and residents. Erikson described eight stages of human development, beginning in infancy and continuing into the geriatric period, each with new challenges and opportunities for growth throughout the life cycle [1]. Of particular importance for medical training are the stages he called Identity vs. Identity Diffusion, which is generally associated with late adolescence, and Generativity vs. Stagnation, a stage that follows young adulthood and is associated with decreased focus on the self and a corresponding increased attention to helping others.

The first of these stages can be applied to medical students and residents, who are essentially in an adolescent stage of professional development with as yet unrealized career aspirations and drive for mastery of the physician role. For them, each faculty member's professional style becomes a potential model during periods of learning. Always be aware of this readiness on the part of learners to take on aspects of your practice patterns, style of interaction with patients, and ways of conceptualizing a case. What the academic physician tries to teach explicitly will be totally overshadowed by what trainees see him or her actually doing.

Over the course of training, particularly for residents, physicians will move into the next Eriksonian stage that defines their generativity. The supervisor will have traversed his or her own identity stages—one hopes—and will embody the generative stage of academic life—providing clinical care, creating new knowledge, and passing on hard-won experience and clinical wisdom to a new generation of doctors. Most academic physicians come to understand that a valuable aspect of work with inquisitive trainees is the accompanying inoculation against professional stagnation. Teaching will force the academic physician to confront his or her biases and to articulate, refine, and expand his or her knowledge base. It is good to enjoy those qualities; as a supervisor it is essential to model, encourage, and reward them in trainees.

What Do Trainees Value in a Clinical Supervisor?

Better than a thousand days of diligent study is one day with a great teacher.

Japanese proverb

Although academic faculty may feel that scholarly activity comprises a substantial portion of their careers, residents do not place a high premium on their supervisors' publication records [2]. Indeed, supervisors with heavy time commitments to research or administration at the expense of their clinical assignments tend to receive low marks from trainees left to fend for themselves in the front lines of care. Few things are more frustrating to a frightened intern than not being able to reach a supervisor who is unavailable because of laboratory commitments or an administrative meeting.

Nor is being liked an adequate measure of teaching success. There is, after all, a body of competencies for each specialty, much of which is imparted in the clinical setting; an attending who strives to be liked at the expense of preparing medical students and residents to pass licensing and specialty board exams is doing the trainee no favor. Nonetheless, the well-regarded attending has the advantage of being a more palatable object of identification for the trainees who work closely with him or her. And since we all function within a range of traits, attitudes, and styles that we can attenuate or exaggerate, it is useful to look at what attributes are valued by students and residents.

A multisite survey of internal medicine residents found that excellent teachers outscored other faculty on time spent with residents, enjoyment of teaching, and importance imputed to giving in-depth feedback and building relationships with house officers [3]. This study added to previous reports that emphasized the need for teaching faculty to display compassion, integrity, humor, and teaching skills. A more recent meta-analysis concluded that such qualities as enthusiasm and support of learners are as crucial to clinical education as the "cognitive" elements of teaching [4]. Importantly, these are not all inherent personal qualities but, rather, characteristics that can be developed and nurtured in an environment that supports good teaching. Interestingly, one family medicine study found that residents and faculty did not necessarily agree on all of the elements of good teaching: residents valued support of their autonomy highly and the need for the supervisor to be a role model less so, while the opposite was true for the faculty [2]. One lesson from this may be that faculty should be more humble in their certitude that their students are eager to emulate them. Nonetheless, just as occurs in the parent–child relationship, both our fine qualities as physicians and our less admirable characteristics are likely to be replicated in our trainees.

Table 8.1 Characteristics of supervisors valued by medical students and residents

Medical students	Residents
• Patient, approachable	• Highly knowledgeable
• Keeps students actively involved	• Respects residents' wishes for autonomy while providing support
• Gives direct feedback	• Appears to love his/her work
• Cares that students learn	• Teaches how to take care of difficult patients
• Shows skill, knowledge, and compassion	• Dedicated to teaching
• Takes time to teach	• Good rapport with patients
• Holds small interactive teaching sessions	• Helpful with time management
• Enjoys teaching	• Makes evidence-based decisions
• Provides structure and clear expectations	• Gives constructive feedback
• Values student input in care of patients	

Finally, it should go without saying that no trainee will flourish in an atmosphere of humiliation, abuse, or belittling and that attending faculty should always model thoughtful, sincere, and encouraging interactions with all learners. Unfortunately, inappropriate behavior by clinical supervisors is common throughout medical training [5, 6]. Such behavior destroys the learning environment, perpetuates the malignant myth that angry outbursts and abusive interactions by faculty are both tolerated and expected, and has an immediate negative effect on patient care [7]. Credentialing bodies for both medical schools and residency programs specify that professionalism in supervisory relationships is essential to a healthy learning environment. Trainees at all levels watch how their supervisors model compassion toward patients. They will inevitably notice if the faculty member interacts effectively and respectfully with an interdisciplinary medical team. Supervisors do well to model appropriate, constructive interactions, to actively watch that their trainees do the same, and to give them feedback on how they are doing (Table 8.1).

Individualizing Teaching to the Resident and Student

Clinical supervisors can learn much from the teaching styles of experts in other fields. The distinguished Julliard violin professor Dorothy Delay, teacher to Itzhak Perlman, Midori, and Sarah Chang, was renowned for her ability to prepare even the most accomplished musicians for the concert stage. In Delay's preparation of one student for performance of a violin concerto with orchestra, not only did she remind her student to "tune sharp to the oboe" so that the violin sound would cut through the heavy orchestra, but she also encouraged the student to free her hair from the restrictive ponytail preferred by this young student's mother. "You mean, I don't need to pull my hair from my face?" the student asked incredulously and was met by Delay's response, "Oh, Heavens, no! If you've got it, flaunt it. You'll excite your audience that way." Although this interaction can be analyzed at multiple levels, Delay's qualities of enthusiasm and engagement are unmistakable. Beginning with a piece of advice that is counterintuitive (departing from being "in tune"), Delay proceeded to offer— indeed, insert—herself as an alternative parental figure who licensed the student to graduate from the violin playing of a late adolescent into full-fledged adult performance [8].

Just as Delay recognized where her student was on the developmental trajectory toward mastery of violin performance in all its aspects, so clinical supervisors should seek to understand the developmental stage of their trainees and challenge them to move to the next level. At its most basic, this requires the academic physician to be aware of the year of training, prior months in the setting, and other experiences that the resident may have had. It also requires sensitivity to the trainee's skill development in the fundamentals of interacting with patients, guiding an interview, and conducting an examination, along with the higher order tasks of formulating a differential diagnosis and individualizing a treatment plan. The physician's capacity to perceive where residents are on this continuum, to detect their unique strengths and weaknesses, and to challenge them to take the next step will define the difference between a tolerable supervisor and a great teacher.

Supervision in the Hospital Setting

It is easily argued that nothing can match the learning opportunities for trainees of a fine teaching hospital. Inpatient medicine — with its acuity, volume of patients, extent and range of pathology, and fast pace — is a proving ground for early-career doctors and the perfect teaching setting for those new to clinical practice. In fact, when many of us reflect back on formative experiences and relationships from medical school and residency, our thoughts turn to hospitals where we trained, with memories of long days and nights on the wards, our first exposure to surgery, and our mentoring by vividly recalled senior residents and faculty who seemed so skillful with these very ill patients.

This is not to say that the hospital setting does not have its challenges for teaching; the noise and bustle, the lack of privacy (and comfortable seating) on rounds, and the constant competing demands on time all contrast with the relative quietude of the outpatient clinic. The academic physician may find that it takes more creativity to deal with the special circumstances of teaching in the hospital; for example, the centrality of the clinical rounds in hospital care poses the challenge of simultaneously teaching residents and students at greatly varying levels of experience and knowledge. Even experienced academic hospital faculty members view with admiration those colleagues who can keep both early-stage medical students and advanced residents and fellows interested and engaged.

Despite the difficulties inherent in hospital-based teaching, you will inevitably come to view bringing your trainees to the point where they can comfortably manage complicated hospital patients as a measure of the success of your efforts. If your residents can take care of the very ill, they will have confidence in themselves as they go forth in their careers. Your goal for them is the achievement of the physician quality that Osler famously termed "Aequanimitas" [9] and that Hemingway described as "grace under pressure." The hospital setting — with its volume, pace, and opportunity for repeated encounters with related disease states and clinical situations — can serve as a proving ground for late-stage residents in their final stages of training, much like a road test on a busy highway. And your residents, while gaining this mastery, will have the added reassurance (and safety) of knowing that a supervisor who knows the patient well is readily at hand. Finally, one of the beauties of hospital-based learning resides in the time-honored structure of medical teams, which allows the more senior trainees to engage the earlier stage learners in teaching moments. The corollary to this for supervisors is that teaching not only involves the imparting of specific clinical knowledge but should also include pedagogic skills as a competency for everyone on the medical team.

Adjusting Teaching to the Level of the Learner

As their teacher, it is the academic physician's responsibility to gain some idea of where his or her students are in their developmental trajectory. Some will be more advanced in their progression, and they can accordingly be granted more responsibility for independent decision-making. A useful practice of effective supervisors is to meet individually with each resident and student at the beginning of their rotations to review their personal goals for the upcoming weeks. Periodic check-ins with the trainees for updates will allow the supervisor to track their progress. It is likewise important to develop tactful ways of telling trainees that they are off-track with regard to their stated goals (or the department's goals for them). For instance, some variation on the following phrasing may be useful: "The people in our field who do this really well look to be able to do X at your point in training. Here is what I think you would need to do to get to that level." Suggestions could involve more reading, practice at a procedure, observation by the attending, and so on.

Thus supervision must be adjusted to the clinical maturity of the trainees. For instance, the learning priorities of medical students differ from those of more advanced residents. Medical students and junior residents can easily feel ignored on hospital rounds, where the discussions are often pitched at the senior residents and where much attention must be directed toward completing the necessary work of caring for patients. Early trainees thrive when they feel acknowledged and, even more so, when they see themselves as needed and as making some real contribution to overall patient care. Meaningful roles for the least experienced members of the team are thus essential to their learning.

One of the talents hospital supervisors must cultivate is the ability to keep all levels of learners engaged in the treatment team. In one study at a teaching hospital, third-year medical students were directed to track thousands of teaching encounters with their faculty supervisors [10]. These students saw high-quality teaching as including the following: mini-lectures from the attending; encouragement for them to give short presentations on inpatient topics; bedside teaching; instruction in reading X-rays and EKGs; and feedback on their physical exams, presentations, documentation, and differential diagnosis skills. These results make intuitive sense; junior-level trainees are building basic competencies and are not ready for the nuances of clinical care. They need to feel the pride and mastery of discerning an infiltrate on a chest film or recognizing Wolff–Parkinson–White syndrome on an EKG for the first time with a real patient. To supplement clinical teaching, novice learners can be directed to secondary sources such as review articles, textbooks, or Internet-based resources. Early-stage trainees can become flustered if presented with material that is too complex and need some "yes/no" information. In confronting a particular clinical situation or disease state, they should be encouraged to go through one pathway in their thought process as opposed to the complex decision tree/algorithm of the more advanced resident.

Hospital supervision of more advanced residents will shift toward deeper diagnostic understanding and greater sophistication in treatment choices, emphasizing the most current primary literature and use of treatment algorithms for complex clinical situations. Residents approaching graduation need to be able to sift through complex clinical information and treatment options. The goal of supervision for these residents is to increase their ability to prioritize the stages of a hospital workup, gain comfort with uncertainty, and avoid the problems of premature closure in their thinking and problem-solving.

Models of Hospital-Based Supervision

Teaching and learning are one shared endeavor, and great teachers inspire learners through a mutually-interactive process that informs and creates community.

Laura Weiss Roberts [11]

Today's trainees, who often have been raised to offer their elders more bemused tolerance than unquestioning respect, appreciate an approach that acknowledges their talents and fosters their autonomy. They seek to be part of a learning community to which they contribute as well as from which they draw. The apprenticeship model of clinical training, founded on the notion of a novice–master relationship in which the senior physician imparts knowledge and praxis to the "empty vessel" learner [12], is a tempting formula for the hospital setting. The patients are so ill, the time-pressure so intense, and the potential for error so lurkingly present that the supervisor can easily lapse into a "this is the way it is done" style of teaching. But although the urgencies of hospital medicine may sometimes call for this directive mode, residents appear to be asking for a more subtle form of instruction that could be defined as "guided autonomy," in which they are increasingly allowed to make clinical decisions while knowing that the supervisor is present, active, and involved.

It is helpful to consider what has been gathered from actual observations of pedagogic styles in a hospital setting. In one study in a Swedish teaching hospital [13], faculty members were observed during clinical rounds and other teaching activities using a variety of forms of teaching that can be categorized as follows:

- *Demonstrating*—The supervisor shows the trainee how to act, assess, view, perceive, and so on.
- *Piloting*—The supervisor focuses on a specific goal using directives without discussion or exploration of the trainee's understanding. This mode is resorted to often with specific tasks, such as ordering fluids: how much, what type, and how quickly.
- *Lecturing*—The supervisor notes a relative lack of knowledge in certain area and offers information regarding the illness, guiding principles and strategies of treatment, and even how to act and communicate with patients.

- *Intervening*—The supervisor interrupts the trainee's interaction and simply takes over the task or the interview. This authoritarian approach can lead the trainee to feel undermined or undervalued, or it may free the trainee from a difficult interaction with a patient or a family.
- *Prompting*—The supervisor directs the trainee toward a correct answer. For example, when a student on rounds looks puzzled as to whether a wound is healing, the attending may whisper, "It looks fine." This can help the trainee establish benchmarks for some clinical phenomena and allows the trainee to save face in front of the patient.
- *Questioning*—The supervisor uses questions to activate discussion, solicits the learner's reasoning process, and offers alternatives. This method can both assess and expand the trainee's knowledge base.
- *Supplementing*—The supervisor adds further clarifying questions and interventions to the trainee's clinical interview or exam. This method works best when trainees signal that they are stuck.

Noticeable in this list is a continuum from attending-focused to learner-focused interactions, but the preponderance of directive teaching is disappointing. In a busy hospital environment—with the exigencies of caring for patients—it is all too easy to intervene with and direct trainees. Indeed, time constraints alone militate against frequent use of Socratic questioning during busy hospital rounds. Nonetheless, those hospital supervisors who take the trouble to examine the admixture of techniques they are using with trainees may note a need to shift—within their own abilities and comfort—toward the addition of more learner-based interactions. Incorporating learner-centered teaching techniques into the day-to-day training is more likely to engage residents and students toward the sustaining goal of "making understanding possible" while supplementing the more practical aim of transmission of specific knowledge.

A collaborative rather than hierarchical approach to work with trainees is more consistent with generational expectations and will go further toward building a true learning community. This approach involves trainees in the gathering and analysis of clinical data, formulation of a differential diagnosis, and proposal of a treatment plan. It readily facilitates development of both clinical skills and use of evidence-based medicine. Essential elements include the following:

- *Observation*. Provide opportunities for the trainee to watch you gathering history, conducting an examination, or discussing the case with the patient and family. With a subsequent patient, give the trainee the opportunity to practice those skills while you observe.
- *Description*. Ask what the trainee observed during the interview and examination, irrespective of who conducted it. Ask additional questions to guide the trainee toward the observations that you consider most pertinent.
- *Exploration*. Probe for understanding of what the observations mean. Help the trainee differentiate among those that are pathognomic, suggestive, or supportive of a diagnosis. Ask for additional information that the trainee will need to clarify their meaning.
- *Analysis*. Have the trainee put together the history, examination, and other data. Ask for a broad differential diagnosis on the basis of information gathered to this point.
- *Integration*. Determine what outside information from textbooks, review articles, and peer-reviewed research papers can be brought to bear on the case. Find out how much of this information the trainee already knows. Make a focused, specific assignment for the trainee to gather more. Assist the trainee in applying the evidence-based information to this case. Help the trainee generalize the findings in this case to others.
- *Commitment*. Give the trainee the opportunity to make a commitment to a specific diagnosis or brief, rank-ordered differential. Have the trainee propose a specific treatment approach.
- *Reflection*. Ask for a rational justification of the diagnosis and treatment plan. Choose 1 or 2 key assertions that the trainee makes in this process and ask, "How do we know that?" Do not accept "In my clinical experience …" or "That's how my last attending did it" as answers. Insist on evidence in the form of research studies or at least expert guidelines. Help the trainee identify the limits of current knowledge and a rational basis for decision-making beyond those limits.

Table 8.2 Pointers for effective clinical teaching

- Use case-based teaching rather than lecturing
- Help your trainees set appropriate goals for themselves
- Give timely and appropriate feedback not laced with criticisms
- Use guided questioning to lead the learner through the clinical thought process, e.g., "What are your choices for this situation?" "What are the pros and cons of each choice?"
- Remember that enthusiasm scores highly as a characteristic of supervisors
- Know your learner. Adjust your teaching to the level of training, individual style, strengths, and vulnerabilities of each trainee
- Humor can be a valuable teaching aid, but should not be directed at your trainees or the patients. If your ego can handle it, humor directed at yourself can be refreshingly humanizing
- The quality of your relationships with learners is important—negative emotions hamper the processing of information, while positive emotions foster learning

Not every step of this process needs to be followed with every case, but some parts of it should be done each day. In fact, this is the mental process that expert clinicians (remember, that is you) go through in most clinical encounters. Clinical teaching simply requires that the academic physician make the sequence conscious, explicit, and subject to discussion. Thus trainees will learn not only facts but also the essential process of clinical decision-making, Table 8.2.

Supervision in the Outpatient Clinic

When you teach you throw a pebble into the water and the ripples from that pebble create an endless ring of concentric circles in such a way that you never know when your influence ends.

Glen O. Gabbard [14]

Work as a supervisor in an outpatient clinic has unique rewards not often found in other settings. Done well, the supervisory experience facilitates the growth and independence of the trainee and enhances the professional satisfaction of the supervisor. In the outpatient setting, the resident physician has often rotated through an inpatient service before arrival on the rotation and therefore may have a broader base of experience and a more developed clinical skillset. The goals of the supervisor will vary slightly on the basis of the resident's level of training but will commonly consist of providing the resident with clinical oversight, professional modeling, and career guidance. This section describes the salient goals and responsibilities of the supervisor and the nuances of different supervisory models of supervision for an outpatient clinical setting. It will also present qualities of a supervisor that will help the academic physician to be successful in this role and effective in his or her goals to guide and foster professional growth in the resident physician.

Clinical Supervision and Professional Development

One of the first tasks as an outpatient supervisor is to understand the expectations of the supervisory role in a particular clinical setting. For whom are you responsible? The focus of this chapter is residents, but supervision may also include medical students, physician assistants, nurse practitioners, social workers, and others. What is their level of training? The needs of a recent medical school graduate, a third-year resident new to the outpatient setting, and a seasoned resident nearing graduation are each unique. What are the educational goals of the rotation? The rotation may primarily be an opportunity for the trainee to learn about a specific patient population, a particular treatment technique, or a unique care setting. How much time is allotted for supervision? Some settings expect you to carry a full load of patients and provide oversight to the trainees only as you do so; others want time to be carved out to discuss cases in a more reflective way. What is the duration of the rotation? Clinic assignments may be as short as a few weeks or as long as a year or more. The supervision you provide will be affected by each of these factors. Clarify how supervision of trainees will mesh with your own clinical responsibilities, whether the residents' work will be incorporated into yours or will be in parallel with it. Ensure that whoever is keeping track of your work performance is aware of the assignment and that it is included in your job description.

The next task is to ensure that trainees know what is expected of them. Be specific about the schedule and the tasks they are to perform. Clarify the issues that they may handle independently and those that will require your prior input. Let them know when and where they are to meet you and what you will discuss at those times. Make arrangements for how they will reach you when urgent matters arise and who will be covering that role when you are not available. Finally, review with them the basis on which they will be evaluated during and at the end of the rotation.

Models of Outpatient Supervision

A common model for supervised outpatient care is for the resident to see a patient independently, and then present and discuss the case with the supervisor who is attending in the clinic. This provides an opportunity for the resident to present the history and examination findings and to propose a diagnostic formulation and treatment plan. As the attending physician, you can then see the patient to meet regulatory and billing requirements, but also to gauge how well the trainee gathered the history, performed the physical examination, and translated those data into a reasonable assessment, differential diagnosis, and care plan. In surgical or procedural clinics, supervision may occur in the context of evaluations, operative procedures, or follow-up appointments, and thus may take place in the operating room itself or during procedures in an ambulatory setting. These encounters allow immediate feedback and direction on the procedure that is occurring.

In both of these models, if the resident's work appears sound, your confirmation in the encounter may be sufficient feedback to the resident. In other cases, a subsequent discussion of additional findings, discrepant observations, or alternative views may be appropriate. Good supervision includes your listening to the trainee's perspectives, both to understand where problems are occurring and to remain open to different views. As you become familiar with the resident's strengths and weaknesses, you will be able to anticipate potential problem areas and concerns that might arise for the resident.

This aspect of supervision benefits from regularly structured, face-to-face meetings with the trainee to discuss broader, more conceptual issues than would be appropriate during individual clinic visits or procedures. For example, the resident may have general questions about a disease or a procedure, or may have noticed a pattern across several patients that would not be appropriate to discuss in the supervision of a single case. In many psychiatry programs, residents see most psychotherapy patients outside of attending-supervised clinics and supervision of these cases is provided entirely separately, in scheduled, one-on-one sessions. Although this would not be appropriate for every setting and each clinic has its own constraints in structure, time, and workload, at least some time carved out to allow the trainee to sit and reflect with a faculty member on the work they do together is well worth the investment of time.

Supervision should include attention to the full range of issues that might affect clinical care. Modeling may include your own interactions with patients, colleagues, ancillary staff members, and the resident. The discussion may cover the patient's healthcare beliefs, treatment preferences, and compliance with treatment. The patient's overall safety, both medically and psychiatrically, will always need to be evaluated. Psychosocial issues such as employment concerns, substance abuse or misuse, finances, and available resources are sometimes overlooked, yet can have a major effect on a patient's overall care if they are addressed and managed. Your attention to these issues conveys an important message to the resident about their value.

The resident should be encouraged to communicate with other members of the treatment team caring for that patient. When the team is housed in the same clinic, it is helpful to work with the resident to optimize interactions with the physician assistants, nurses, psychologists, social workers, and others who work collaboratively in the care of the patient. Equally important is communication with outside providers who referred the patient or are otherwise participating in the patient's care. The supervisor is responsible to ensure that this communication occurs, includes the appropriate information, conveys a respectful and collegial tone, and follows all pertinent privacy regulations.

Associated with individual patient encounters are the documentary expectations of medical care, such as clinical notes, care plans, billing codes, insurance reviews, and disability forms. These issues form an inevitable part of clinical care but are rarely discussed, modeled, or reviewed in supervision. The function of this type of supervision is multifactorial. Reading and editing the notes (or at least scanning them for key items) allow you to keep abreast of the resident's caseload and to meet legal and payer requirements. The notes help you gain insight into the trainee's skill with documentation, understanding of diagnostic issues, and medical decision-making. They allow you to reflect on questions, concerns, or ideas about the care of the patient that you will want to discuss with the resident at the next supervision session. They provide a basis for you to work with the resident to develop skills in organization, time management, and prioritization. Feedback on the quality of clinical documentation will contribute to pithy, well-focused, grammatically comprehensible notes that enhance the care of patients, build the trainee's confidence, and earn the respect of collaborative care providers.

Guiding Personal and Career Development

The greatest sign of a success for a teacher...is to be able to say, "The children are now working as if I did not exist."

Maria Montessori

The academic physician can have a significant role in helping the resident identify personal strengths and weaknesses as a clinician. Respect, interest, and flexibility, as well as being genuine, available, and approachable to residents, are important characteristics that help them navigate and be successful in this capacity. Positive feedback and constructive comments are most effective when they are identified and given in a focused and timely manner. Recognizing and discussing these positive factors allow the residents to balance strengths with the constructive criticism that is more commonly brought to their attention during their training experience.

Critical issues from a resident's interactions with patients or staff may be raised as a concern in the clinic. Feedback on the resident's interpersonal style is best provided in a confidential setting, face to face. When discussing such concerns, listen to the resident's view of the situation and how it might be handled. Make specific suggestions that can be readily implemented to correct the problem. Make a follow-up plan to give ongoing feedback on the resident's progress.

Watch carefully for evidence of burnout and depression; it is critical for the supervisor to notice and address such a situation with the resident. This might include a discussion of the problem confidentially, a suggestion for the resident to contact an employee or house officer assistance program, or recommendations for treatment outside the system.

Supervision of senior residents should expand to include discussion of short- and long-term career goals and professional development after residency. It can be extremely helpful to adjust the resident's caseload to reflect the trainee's unique needs and interests. For example, you can help steer certain cases to the resident on the basis of patients' diagnoses, symptom profiles, or treatment needs that may be of specific interest to the trainee. Faculty members are in a position to provide trainees with professional mentoring for their professional activities and career goals. Mentorship includes discussion of the resident's past experiences, current interests, professional objectives, and long-term aspirations. It includes personal sharing of one's own experiences, knowledge, and recommendations related to the resident's specific needs.

Supervisors within the academic setting can provide professional contacts for the resident to establish a network of individuals who can be resources of information on job openings, research opportunities, and specialty meetings. Guidance regarding membership in professional organizations may be useful. The importance of continuing medical education and techniques for meeting licensing and certification requirements are often overlooked in training, yet are critical for the graduating resident, Table 8.3.

Table 8.3 Goals of outpatient supervision

- Provide clinical guidance and oversight for individual cases
- Manage and customize the clinical caseload to ensure the right mix for the resident's educational and career development needs
- Anticipate problems and/or concerns in both the resident's clinical care and personal well-being
- Model professional behavior as a physician and mentor
- Provide career mentoring for senior residents; discuss career goals and steps for development toward them

Direct Observation

Although most often used with novice learners such as medical students, opportunities for residents to observe faculty during routine clinical encounters remain an invaluable tool for supervision in any outpatient setting. In clinics where physical examinations, procedures, and testing are done, the supervisor's experience can be essential to guide the resident in making reliable, effective clinical assessments. As the supervisor models interactions with more difficult patients and higher level examination techniques, he or she may highlight unusual physical findings and demonstrate new procedures directly; this shared experience is perfect material for discussion at the time or in a subsequent session.

Equally important, but too rarely done in clinical settings, is direct observation of a resident conducting an entire patient encounter, an enormously valuable exercise for both the resident and supervisor. This type of observation requires the supervisor to be present but passive as the resident does the full interview and examination and to step out of the room before the final discussion with the patient. The resident may then formally present the case, propose a formulation, and recommend treatment options, just as is done on other occasions. In this case, however, the supervisor has access to the raw data the resident gathered and can comment on the interaction with the patient, the interview process, and other aspects of the patient assessment. As the supervisor returns to make a final treatment plan with the patient, he or she may choose to model some aspects of the interaction to demonstrate teaching points.

These sessions permit the resident to demonstrate interview and examination skills and allow the supervisor to assess what actually happened in the visit, rather than trying to surmise what happened on the basis of the resident's report and the supervisor's subsequent repetition of "key portions" of the examination. The feedback given to residents following these observations has a legitimacy and immediacy not otherwise available and residents benefit from feedback on the interaction itself, as well as on the presentation, diagnostic impression, and plan for the care of the patient. The time required of faculty and anxiety provoked in residents are a small price to pay for the quality of information that is gathered.

Group Supervision

The most common setting for group supervision is within a clinic's team meeting before or after the patient visits. Here, the supervisor's role as team leader includes supervision of one or more residents and other staff involved in the patients' care. Clinics run differently depending on the specialty and patient population, but several elements are likely to be present. Residents are typically expected to present the cases to provide the raw material for discussion, participation of several members of the team is expected, and the supervisor is responsible for final decisions regarding treatment planning. The supervisor may choose to ask questions of those present to probe the depth of their knowledge and to encourage thoughtful analysis or may expound on some aspect of the case, preferably related to the work of the treatment team. It is appropriate to give trainees assignments to seek out additional information on topics that they will report later. This is an ideal time to model professional interactions with the other team members, including such vital skills as how to solicit dissenting opinions, diffuse conflicts, and acknowledge the limits of one's knowledge and experience.

Group supervision is especially useful when the goal is to teach a particular modality of care, such as a specific procedure or therapy technique. Simultaneous work with more than one resident increases clinical exposure for several trainees, covers more cases in a short time, and provides opportunities for peer interaction and input. The structure of such groups varies from as few as 2 to as many as 10 clinicians, along with 1 or 2 facilitators/supervisors. The sessions may occur only a few times or may be ongoing for 6–12 months. For longer training periods, the first sessions may include a didactic introduction and overview of the treatment modality, followed by subsequent sessions in which residents bring their own cases for group discussion. The supervisor role in this case may expand to include didactic teaching along with ongoing guidance and direction for the residents more typical of conventional supervision.

Feedback and Evaluation

The evaluation of residents is described in detail in another chapter of this book. A brief overview of evaluation as it occurs in outpatient clinics will be given here to address issues particularly connected to outpatient supervision. Formative evaluation includes immediate feedback to the resident about a particular situation or a specific issue that requires positive or negative comment. It may be given at any time throughout the rotation and should be a regular feature of interactions. The long duration typical of outpatient supervision makes ongoing assessment and feedback especially important. Formative comments may be brief but should always be specific, prompt, and constructive. Try to identify at least one thing about which to give feedback during every session. Comment on it at the time and make a note in preparation for a future summative evaluation.

More comprehensive summative evaluations may occur at intervals of 1–6 months, but should never be allowed to languish longer than that; for year-long rotations, quarterly summations are ideal. These evaluations should include an overall evaluation of the resident's development of the core competencies of patient care, medical knowledge, interpersonal skills, professionalism (including clinical documentation), adaptation to the clinical setting, improvement with practice, and ability to use supervision appropriately during the rotation. Every aspect of the summative feedback should have been addressed previously with formative comments. There should be no surprises for the resident in the final evaluation.

The academic physician should expect to receive feedback from trainees on his or her performance as a supervisor. The nature of faculty–trainee relationships includes such a steep power differential that most institutions limit feedback to an annual summative assessment, usually compiled from several different trainees to ensure their anonymity. Candid, constructive feedback is essential to continued growth as a supervisor and should be welcomed even when critical.

Conclusion

Clinical supervision is an invaluable tool to educate and guide resident physicians over the course of their training, with many rewards for both the resident and the supervisor. The essential elements are an awareness of who the trainees are, what they know, and what they can do; encouragement of their development through learner-centered interactions; and prompt, focused feedback to guide their growth. The role of mentor and educator takes time, dedication, and effort, but the endeavor holds tremendous value for the resident, and the academic physician will benefit in the process.

Words to the Wise
- Your behavior and quality of character carry a stronger message than anything you say. Make sure you exemplify the highest ideals of the profession.
- Depth of knowledge and academic standing are far less important to trainees than willingness to spend time and build relationships with them, along with compassion, integrity, and humor.
- Adjust your teaching to the level of training and individual strengths and weaknesses of the trainee. Make the effort to find out what those are.
- Give prompt, focused feedback that emphasizes positive achievements and gives direction to address deficiencies.
- Provide career mentoring and monitoring of resident well-being as well as oversight of clinical cases.

Ask Your Mentor or Colleagues
- How do you structure your time and interactions during supervision?
- What questions have you found to be most effective in stimulating discussion with your trainees?
- As you reflect on your experiences as a supervisor, what lessons have you learned?
- What have you enjoyed most about supervision? What has been the greatest challenge?

References

1. Erikson E. Childhood and society. 2nd ed. New York: WW Norton; 1963.
2. Buchel TL, Edwards FD. Characteristics of effective clinical teachers. Fam Med. 2005;37:30–5.
3. Wright SM, Kern DE, Kolodner K, et al. Attributes of excellent attending-physician role models. N Engl J Med. 1998;339:1986–93.
4. Sutkin G, Wagner E, Harris I, Schiffer R. What makes a good clinical teacher in medicine? A review of the literature. Acad Med. 2008;83:452–66.
5. Frank E, Carrera JS, Stratton T, et al. Experiences of belittlement and harassment and their correlates among medical students in the United States: longitudinal survey. BMJ. 2006;333:682.
6. Cook DJ, Liutkus JF, Risdon CL, et al. Residents' experiences of abuse, discrimination and sexual harassment during residency training: McMaster University residency training programs. CMAJ. 1996; 154:1657–65.
7. Mazzocco K, Petitti DB, Fong KT, et al. Surgical team behaviors and patient outcomes. Am J Surg. 2009;197: 678–85.
8. Kransberg-Talvi M. A lesson with Dorothy Delay. Chamber musician todayhttp://chambermusiciantoday.com/blog/posts/A-Lesson-with-Dorothy-DeLay. Accessed 15 Feb 2012.
9. Osler W. Aequanimitas: with other addresses to medical students, nurses and practitioners of medicine. Philadelphia: P. Blakiston's; 1905.
10. Torre DM, Sebastian JL, Simpson DE. Learning activities and high-quality teaching: perceptions of third-year IM clerkship students. Acad Med. 2003; 78:812–4.
11. Roberts LW. Teaching by great teachers. Acad Psychiatry. 2011;35:275–6.
12. Haidet P, Stein HF. The role of the student-teacher relationship in the formation of physicians. J Gen Intern Med. 2006;21:S16–20.
13. Nilsson M, Pennbrant P, Pilhammar E, Wenestam C-G. Pedagogical strategies used in clinical medical education: an observational study. BMC Med Educ. 2010;10:9.
14. Gabbard GO. Why I teach. Acad Psychiatry. 2011;35(5):277–82.

How to Evaluate and Give Feedback

9

Jennifer R. Kogan

A key and critical component of medical education is evaluating learners and providing them with feedback. Evaluation is the process by which the academic physician assesses whether the learner has achieved the goals and objectives outlined by a course or by the clinical rotation or experience. Feedback is the impetus for improving performance. It is a fundamental cornerstone of effective teaching and learning. This chapter focuses on how to assess learners for the purpose of providing feedback. The chapter also reviews some best practices regarding the completion of evaluations.

What Is Feedback?

Feedback can be conceptualized as specific information about a learner's observed performance compared with a standard, given with the intent to improve the learner's performance. This definition highlights several important concepts. First, feedback is based on observed performance. In the classroom setting, this

J.R. Kogan, M.D. (✉)
Department of Medicine, Perelman School of Medicine at the University of Pennsylvania, 3701 Market Street, Philadelphia, PA, USA
e-mail: Jennifer.Kogan@uphs.upenn.edu

© Springer International Publishing Switzerland 2016
L.W. Roberts (ed.), *The Clinician Educator Guidebook*,
DOI 10.1007/978-3-319-27980-0_9

could be a student's ability to apply knowledge to a problem-based learning case. In the clinical setting, feedback may focus on the core clinical skills of history taking, physical exam, interpersonal skills with patients, professionalism, and humanism. Feedback could also focus on the academic physician's observation of learners' skills related to transitions of care, interpersonal interactions with the team, oral case presentations, documentation in the medical record, or problem-solving abilities. Second, the aforementioned definition highlights that the intent of feedback is to help the learner acquire the knowledge, skills, and attitudes to improve. Third, the content of the feedback focuses on the difference in performance between how the learner is doing and a standard. For example, feedback content is about the difference between how a learner does the cardiac exam and best practices for the cardiac exam. Finally, and most important, the aim of feedback is learner improvement. Feedback is meant to be a catalyst for additional learning. It has been said that feedback is really an assessment *for* learning rather than an assessment *of* learning. In this way, the academic physician can think of himself or herself in the role of a coach for learners.

Differences Between Feedback and Evaluation

It is helpful, when thinking about feedback and evaluation, to be clear about the differences between the two. Evaluation is usually summative, meaning that it happens at the end of a defined period of time. It is about past performance, and it conveys a judgment. The purpose of evaluation is to measure a learner's achievement for the purpose of providing a grade or making decisions about progression or for certification. Evaluation is often normative (comparing one learner to other learners), but it is increasingly becoming criterion based (to what degree does the learner meet explicit standards of performance). Evaluation can be high stakes (professional certification) or low stakes (grade on quiz or assignment) or anywhere along that continuum.

In contrast, feedback is formative, meaning that it happens in real time with the intent of helping the learner develop and improve.

Feedback is designed to foster learning. Feedback is about current, rather than past, performance. It is meant to convey information, reinforce strengths, and identify areas in need of improvement, "before it counts."

Types of Feedback

Feedback can further be divided into "micro-feedback" and "macro-feedback."

Micro-Feedback

Micro-, or brief, feedback is feedback in the moment. As its name suggests, it is brief, approximately 1–2 min in duration. It can be thought of as feedback nuggets. Ideally, because it is so brief, micro-feedback can, and should, be frequent (i.e., daily). An example of micro-feedback would be, "*Let me show you a better way to assess the jugular venous pressure on this patient.*" Often, this type of feedback is not recognized by the learner. Therefore, it is helpful to start micro-feedback by telling the learner that one is about to give feedback. For example, "*Let me give you some feedback about how you checked the jugular venous pressure.*"

Macro-Feedback

Macro-feedback is usually more formal. Examples of macro-feedback include sitting down with a learner after observing his or her history and physical exam or after listening to a patient or topic presentation. Macro-feedback also includes mid-rotation or mid-course feedback. Macro-feedback tends to be a sit-down conversation. It lasts longer than micro-feedback, for example 5–20 min. It tends to cover a broader array of skills and competencies. Macro-feedback tends to occur less frequently, but it is usually a more detailed conversation.

Why Is Feedback Important in Academic Medicine?

Feedback is essential in medical education so that learners can improve. To improve, learners need external information about how they are doing. This is particularly true because self-assessment, defined as an individual's assessment of personal performance or skill, is often inaccurate. Given the inaccuracy of self- assessment, self-assessment must be externally informed. This means that a learner must use not only internal data but also external data to generate an appraisal of his or her own ability.

To better understand this concept, it may be helpful to think about an analogy outside of medicine. Imagine a student who is learning to play the piano. Imagine that the student plays a piece of music. After playing, she identifies what she believes she did well and what she needs to work on. Imagine that the student never plays the piece for her teacher or someone more skilled than she. Without this external input, just how much better could the student get? How likely is it that she will be able to identify and then correct all of her mistakes?

Therefore, feedback is essential for learners. It helps learners identify their strengths and weaknesses without academic penalty. Feedback facilitates learning by providing learners with the information they need to practice and enhance their knowledge and skills. As such, feedback serves as a stimulus for professional growth. As we will see shortly, feedback should be about agreed-upon goals. Therefore, feedback clarifies the expectations of the learner.

Not only is feedback important for learners, but it is also important for teachers. Feedback done well is strongly associated with teaching ratings. Additionally, being proactive about giving feedback helps the teacher to really be cognizant of the learners' progress and their accomplishments, or lack thereof. It also provides the teacher with an opportunity to modify a course or teaching to provide more learner-centered education. That is, by understanding where the learner is, and what it is he or she needs, the teacher has an opportunity to tailor the teaching methods to the individual learners and their current abilities.

Feedback has also taken on heightened importance in this era of competency-based medical education. The focus of training and assessment is increasingly on teaching and assessing competence by documentation of achievement of the milestones. This requires ongoing assessment of trainees, with formative feedback, to ensure progression to clinical competence.

Medical Education Without Feedback

What happens when learners do not get feedback? Many problems arise. Without feedback there are missed learning opportunities. Without positive feedback, good practice is not reinforced. Without negative feedback, poor performance goes uncorrected, medical learning is incomplete, a path to improvement is not identified, and full potential may not be realized. Think back to the example of the piano student. Imagine that the student has a teacher, but the teacher only listens to the student play without ever providing any suggestions for how she might play differently. Imagine how the student's ultimate proficiency would plateau. Imagine an athlete who never is told by his coach how to get better. How good can that athlete get?

An additional problem arises when learners do not get feedback. Without feedback, learners may uphold uncorrected, inaccurate perceptions of their performance. That is, without feedback, learners may assume that they are doing a good job when, in fact, they are not. In these situations, it is not uncommon that learners will be surprised and disappointed with their final evaluations because they will think they were "doing a good job" since they received no information to the contrary. This situation can also lead to learner frustration with final evaluations because the learner, in the absence of feedback, will not feel that he or she had sufficient opportunity to improve in areas identified as needing improvement. Not uncommonly, students and residents will say that had they known there was an area of concern, they would have worked on it or changed their behaviors or attitudes. Not being given that opportunity to improve, secondary to a lack of feedback, is perceived to be unfair.

There is yet another consequence when learners do not get feedback. Without feedback, many learners will start feeling insecure about their abilities, particularly when there is no reinforcing feedback. The absence of feedback can make learners anxious and nervous because they have no sense of how they are doing and they have no idea of what they need to do to get better.

Barriers to Giving Feedback

Despite its importance, many learners are dissatisfied with the feedback that they receive, in terms of its quantity, frequency, and perceived quality. The reality is that many teachers feel uncomfortable giving feedback, and most have never had training in how to do it. In addition to a lack of training in best feedback practices, there are many additional reasons that high-quality feedback does not happen. Lack of time is frequently identified as one of the biggest barriers to giving feedback. Faculty may feel that there is inadequate time to give feedback when there are competing expectations for clinical productivity, research, scholarship, and administrative functions. In the past decade, the length of time that a teacher works with a learner, particularly in the clinical setting, has been markedly abbreviated (i.e., 1- or 2-week attending rotations). The absence of longer, more longitudinal interactions with a learner can effect feedback in multiple ways. First, faculty may feel like they have insufficient information about a learner's performance to provide feedback. Second, lack of an established learner/faculty relationship can leave faculty more uncomfortable giving feedback because they are less familiar with how a particular learner might best respond to feedback.

A very real barrier to giving feedback is providing negative feedback. Even when given constructively, there are many reasons why giving negative feedback is hard. Teachers are often concerned about undesirable consequences for the learner, such as undermining the learner's self-esteem. Faculty may worry that giving negative feedback will jeopardize the relationship they have with the trainee. Giving negative feedback may feel like giving bad news, and one may be overly negative or critical communicating this information.

What also makes feedback challenging is that it often must be delivered within the context of a flawed learner self-assessment. Feedback never occurs in a vacuum. It is given in the context of a learner's own impressions of his or her ability. The perceived value of feedback depends on the ease to which it is reconciled with the learner's self-assessment.

In addition to negative consequences for the learner, many faculty may also worry about the undesirable consequences of giving negative feedback for them as a teacher. For example, faculty may worry that giving negative feedback to a learner will reflect poorly on them as a teacher. They may be concerned that the learner will, in turn, evaluate them poorly. Faculty may then worry about the effect of these evaluations on their own advancement and promotion.

Characteristics of Effective Feedback

Knowing how to give feedback well is important to maximally help the learner. Again, feedback given well is a key catalyst to learning. Additionally, it is important to give feedback well, since feedback also has the potential to harm. For example, negative feedback, if not given correctly, can demotivate learners and actually lead to deterioration in their performance. What follows, then, are some essential characteristics of effective feedback. These characteristics, along with examples, are summarized in Table 9.1.

- *Give feedback frequently.* Think of feedback as a normal daily component of any teacher–student interaction. Up front, let the learner know that you give feedback often. You can even let your learners know early on that "no one is perfect" and "mistakes are expected" and that "everyone is here to learn." This helps to establish the expectation of daily, frequent feedback and can promote a culture that feedback is for the sake of learning. Your frequent, daily feedback or feedback nuggets (i.e., micro-feedback) then sets the stage for more comprehensive, macro-feedback later.
- *Focus feedback on agreed-upon goals.* As a teacher it is always important to set goals for your learners. You can create goals

Table 9.1 Characteristics of effective feedback and examples

Feedback characteristic	Examples
Establish the expectation of frequent feedback	*"This week, I hope to give you a lot of feedback so that I can really help you to be the best doctor you can be"*
Make feedback about specific goals, both yours and the learners	*"This week, I would like for you to focus on making your patient presentations more hypothesis driven"*
	"What do you hope to get out of this course or rotation?"
	"What skills do you want to focus on this week?"
Make feedback timely	
Signpost your feedback	*"I am going to give you a little feedback now"*
	"I want to give you a little feedback on …"
	"Let me give you some feedback about …"
Start with the learner's self-assessment	*"How do you think that went?"*
	"How do you think things are going?"
	"What are you trying to work on?"
	"What do you want feedback about?"
Be specific	*"You paused often when delivering the bad news and you responded to the patient's emotion. That was really well done"* NOT *"You did a great job delivering the news"*
	"Your problem list was missing important alternative diagnoses" NOT *"Your write-up was inadequate"*
Provide positive feedback	*"Your decision to assess the patient's gait was very important for understanding potential causes for falls"*
Provide constructive feedback about areas requiring improvement	*"The history would have been more organized if you had set an agenda with the patient prior to exploring her chief complaint"*
Prioritize feedback	
Make feedback descriptive, not evaluative	*"I thought you could have demonstrated more empathy by pausing more to listen to the patient"* NOT *"You are un-empathic and cold-hearted"*
	"I thought that a key part of the history, his occupational exposure, was omitted" NOT *"Your history was totally inadequate"*
Discuss a specific action plan	*"Focus your reading on how to distinguish systolic from diastolic murmurs"* NOT *"Read more"*
	"Practice your presentations out loud at least twice before presenting to the attending" NOT *"Work on your presentations"*

about your course, lecture, or rotation. You can set learning goals for the week, a given day, or even a specific patient encounter. The best goals are those that are specific, clear, and concise. In addition to articulating your goals, you also should have your learners identify their learning goals too. Getting your learners to set goals is essential so that they then become active participants in the learning process by reflecting on their learning needs. In fact, the ability to frequently ask the learner what he or she desires from a teaching interaction and working with the learner to establish mutually agreed-upon goals and objectives has been associated with a proficiency in feedback skills. Once you and the learner have identified learning goals, prioritize them. Sometimes you will need to negotiate which goals to focus on. Again, the purpose of identifying goals is that this becomes the platform upon which your feedback is based. By establishing the goals, you know what to focus your observations on. Your learners will also be clear about the criteria against which their performance will be assessed. As such, it is beneficial, up front, to make sure that your learner shares with you an understanding of what your conception of good performance looks like.

- *Make feedback timely.* Feedback is best when given close to the observed activity. However, there are exceptions to this rule. Feedback given to a sleep-deprived trainee is often met with an emotional response (crying). Learners who are fatigued cannot rationally process and integrate constructive feedback. In these situations, it is often best to delay the feedback. Similarly, it is often necessary to delay feedback after a medical error because overwhelming emotions (both yours and the learners) can make it hard to both give and receive feedback.
- *Give feedback in a quiet place.* Feedback should ideally be given in a quiet, private location. This is particularly important for macro-feedback. Micro- or brief feedback is often given in the moment.
- *Signpost your feedback.* Feedback is often not recognized by learners as feedback. Therefore, it is helpful to signpost your feedback so that the learner knows it is coming and will be more likely to recognize it.

- *Start by asking for your learner's self-assessment.* There are many reasons why asking the learner for his or her own assessment is essential. First, it makes feedback an interactive conversation rather than a one-way transfer of information. Second, it helps you to assess the learner's level of insight. A self-assessment that is very different from your impression of performance is important to recognize in advance of giving feedback. Imagine giving feedback when the learner thinks his or her performance was outstanding at the same time that you believe there are significant deficiencies. That conversation will be very different from one in which the learner accurately recognizes areas of difficulty. By asking the learner to self-assess, you are also helping the learner to become better at reflection, an important skill in lifelong learning and the self-regulated profession of medicine.
- *Be specific.* Feedback should be detailed and specific. It is less helpful to provide generalities of performance (i.e., "*You did a great job.*"). Although telling someone he or she did a great job makes the learner feel good, it will not help the learner advance his or her knowledge, skills, and attitudes. Feedback must describe specific behaviors.
- *Reinforce the positives.* It is important to reinforce what learners are doing well. This is more than an exercise in making the learner feel good or offering generic praise. Positive feedback should reinforce the knowledge, attitudes, or skills that you want the learner to continue to demonstrate. Ideally, focus this positive feedback on unique positive attributes of the learner, areas in which performance exceeds peers, or strengths observed during challenging or difficult circumstances (i.e., a difficult topic or a challenging clinical encounter).
- *Constructively give feedback about areas requiring improvement.* If learners are to advance in their knowledge, skills, and attitudes and improve their competence or expertise in a given domain, they need to know what requires improvement. They need to know what needs work and what they need to do better on the next time.
- *Focus feedback on directly observable behaviors.* Learners may discount feedback if they believe that the teacher does not have

an accurate knowledge of their performance. Particularly as it relates to clinical skills, there is evidence that medical students and residents are observed relatively infrequently while performing many key clinical activities. Therefore, if you want to provide feedback about core clinical skills such as information gathering (history taking and physical exam), information transfer (counseling and communication of a plan), and interpersonal skills with patients and with the team, you must identify ways to be present during those activities (i.e., watching your learner with a patient; watching your learner with the team). The more you observe patient-related activities, the more likely the trainee will view you as having accurate knowledge of his or her performance. This is important to increase the learner's receptiveness to feedback.

- *Prioritize your feedback.* If you offer too much feedback at a single time, it will be difficult for the learner to process it all. If feedback is not processed, it cannot be integrated and used. Too much feedback at one time can leave the learner feeling overwhelmed and even demoralized. Therefore, you need to make decisions about how you will prioritize the feedback you want to give. Limit your constructive feedback to no more than 2–3 elements.

- *Make feedback descriptive not evaluative.* The purpose of feedback is to improve a learner's competence, not to intentionally make the learner feel bad. Therefore, you need to keep the feedback about the performance not the person. Phrasing feedback nonjudgmentally is more likely to make the feedback more acceptable and palatable to the trainee. Using the word "I" instead of "you" reinforces that what you say is your perception and can make feedback sound less accusatory.

- *Include an action plan.* Feedback without specific suggestions for how the learner can narrow the gap between current and expected or desired performance falls short in effectiveness. All feedback should have an action plan. An action plan includes the specific recommendations for how the learner will get from point A to point B. It provides information for how the learner can narrow the aforementioned gap so that he or she can advance. Action plans can be thought of as an intervention. It should provide helpful suggestions for what should the learner needs to do to acquire needed skills. As with feedback, action plans are best when they are detailed and specific.

- *Follow-up with the learner.* Because the goal of feedback is to help the learner improve, whenever possible, you should try to observe the learner again to see if your feedback was incorporated. Even if you do not have an opportunity to work with the learner again, it is still important to give feedback. In situations where you will not work with the learner again, think about how you could encourage the trainee to seek additional feedback about the identified skill area with his or her next supervisor.
- *Create a climate of trust and comfort for the learner.* You need to be giving feedback in the context of wanting to help the learner. Credible feedback is based on the perception of genuine concern for the learner and a relationship of mutual respect. Part of giving feedback is also checking your own intentions before giving feedback. Sometimes you may feel angry or upset with the learner. These feelings need to be in-check before you give feedback, because feedback really needs to come from a place of wanting to help the trainee improve.

Creating a climate of trust and comfort also means paying attention to the learner's emotional response to feedback. When you perceive such a response, you need to be ready to discuss it.

Another strategy for creating a climate of trust is to make feedback bidirectional. Learners are more likely to appreciate feedback if you also indicate early on that you welcome, expect, and also want feedback from the learner.

Approaches to Giving Feedback

It is important to know that simple do and do not rules for giving feedback underestimate the complexity inherent in how feedback should be delivered. The effectiveness of any feedback approach depends extensively on the context in which the feedback is being delivered and received. Therefore, as you think about how you want to give feedback, you need to recognize that you will need to have an inherent flexibility in your feedback approach that is based on the learner, the content of the feedback, and the context in which you are giving it.

The Feedback Sandwich

One of the most common approaches for giving feedback that people talk about is the "feedback sandwich." The feedback sandwich involves giving positive feedback first so that the trainee is receptive to what comes next. Next comes the negative feedback, the "meat of the sandwich." This is followed by additional positive feedback. Although easy to remember, there are some limitations to this approach. First, sandwiching the negative feedback may be more about the preservation of learner self-esteem. Second, the feedback sandwich quickly becomes predictable for the learner who hears the positive and then is waiting for the "but." Third, the "but" between the positive and constructive feedback often leads the learner to discount the positive feedback. And finally, this approach fails to promote a dialogue or conversation about performance since the teacher is doing all of the talking. It does not remind the teacher to get a self-assessment or end feedback with an action plan.

A Six-Step Approach

Feedback probably works best when it is a conversation between you and the learner, rather than a one-directional flow of information from you to the learner. The following six-step approach helps promote a "feedback conversation." This approach emphasizes seeking and responding to the learner's self-assessment and identifying an action plan which catalyzes future learning. It requires you to be an active listener who can reflect back what you hear. The six-step approach, along with examples, is summarized in Fig. 9.1.

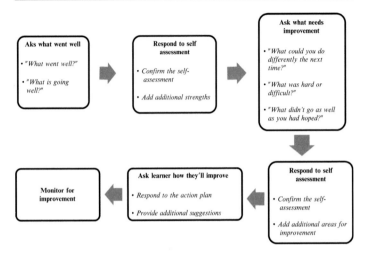

Fig. 9.1 A six-step approach to giving feedback

Step 1. Get the learner's self-assessment about what was good about his or her performance.

Step 2. Respond to the self-assessment by identifying the strengths you agree with and any other strengths about which you want to elaborate.

Step 3. Get the learner's self-assessment about what could have been improved. This step and the next are truly the heart of the feedback conversation. It is these two steps where a significant proportion of the feedback time should be spent.

Step 4. Respond to the learner's self-assessment about what needed improvement. Identify what you agree with and review additional areas needing improvement.

Step 5. Ask the learner to reflect on what they might do to improve. Ask them to identify an action plan. Elaborate on the learner's response, correct it, and add to it as needed. It is very important at this point to make sure that your learner understands what he or she needs to work on and how he or she will do so.

Step 6. Monitor for improvement. Make a commitment to monitoring for improvement together. If you will not have an opportunity to work with the learner again, help the learner to identify ways to find out if he or she has successfully improved.

Difficult Feedback Situations

There are certain situations in which feedback is particularly difficult to give. Examples include giving feedback to a learner who has poor interpersonal skills or has issues with professionalism, giving feedback to the learner who really lacks insight into his or her performance, or giving feedback to the learner who is not receptive to feedback. Often, these situations involve learners who will require remediation, and this is when the academic physician will want to involve the appropriate individuals in the medical school or the course, clerkship, residency, or fellowship directors.

Feedback About Professionalism and Interpersonal Skills

Many faculty find it particularly difficult to give feedback about deficiencies in a learner's professionalism or interpersonal skills because it often feels as though that feedback is about the learner's character or personality. It may feel more subjective and also more resistant to remediation. Nevertheless, addressing lapses in professionalism or interpersonal skills is just as important as addressing a deficient fund of knowledge.

The principles of effective feedback that have been previously described still apply. When giving feedback about professionalism or interpersonal skills, it is especially important to begin by seeking out the learner's self-assessment. For example, when there are concerns about communication skills one might ask, *"How do you feel like you have been interacting with the team?"* or *"How have your interactions with your patients been?"* As with all feedback, it is especially important to be descriptive, not evaluative, describing behaviors, not the person. Using "I" statements instead of "you" statements will also make the feedback less accusatory. When providing feedback about these competencies, it can be helpful to start by saying *"The perception is that ...."* For example, one might say, *"The perception is that you have seemed very short with the nurses."* Phrasing feedback this way can make its delivery easier because the learner cannot argue with a perception.

Feedback to the Learner Who Lacks Insight or Is Not Receptive

It is very challenging to give feedback to a learner who is unaware of his or her limitations or weaknesses (i.e., unconscious incompetence). The learner who lacks insight may be resistant to discussing the problem at hand, may not accept ownership or responsibility for his or her weaknesses, and may find excuses for his or her actions by blaming others or the system. Such a learner will often rationalize and/or externalize negative outcomes and therefore be resistant to getting feedback.

When giving feedback to a learner who lacks insight, try to focus the conversation on further elaborating the problem. Try to encourage additional self-assessment from the learner. Rereview expectations and try to address denial through education. The goal is to try to get the learner to identify the discrepancy between his or her present performance and the expectations or the professional standard.

Although it is difficult to receive negative feedback, most learners will be receptive because they wish to improve. However, some learners are simply not receptive to feedback. Lack of receptivity may be detected through verbal and nonverbal cues from the learner. When a learner is not receptive to feedback, it is incumbent on the academic physician to figure out why. Again, this is when one should be contacting the course director, school administration, or the training director (e.g., fellowship or program director). There is often a reason for a learner's lack of receptivity to feedback, which can be remembered by the four Ds: distraction, drugs, depression, and diagnosis. Sometimes learners are not receptive because they are distracted by issues outside of work, such as problems in a relationship, ill family members, or financial stressors. An underlying problem with substance abuse should be considered, particularly when a learner is erratic in behavior or does not seem to change behavior when expectations are explicitly set. A depressed learner also will have difficulty integrating feedback, as will a learner with any other type of personality disorder or psychiatric or medical diagnosis.

A Few Tips About Evaluation

As described earlier, evaluation is a summative assessment that occurs at the end of the time one is working with the learner. It summarizes whether the learner achieved predetermined goals and expectations. Learners can be evaluated in many ways, such as written examinations, oral exams, clinical skills exams, and 360° evaluations. The most common type of assessment the academic physician will likely be asked to complete is an end-of-course, end-of-clerkship, or end-of-rotation evaluation of the learner. The criteria for assessment and the structure of the assessment form will differ from institution to institution and may also vary within the institution. What follows, therefore, are some general recommendations about how to approach completing these evaluations.

- *Familiarize yourself with the assessment form before working with the learner.* It is very important that you know what the assessment form looks like before you work with the learner. Reviewing the evaluation form tells you what competencies you will be asked to assess and will inform what types of observations you will need to make of the learner. For example, if competence in the physical exam is to be evaluated, it is incumbent upon you to figure out how to observe the learner doing a physical exam. You also must observe the learner's physical exam several times to ensure that your evaluation is reliable. Nothing frustrates a learner more than reading an evaluation when the teacher or supervisor has not directly observed the item to be assessed.
- *Do not evaluate items you have not had the opportunity to observe.* Most evaluation forms have an option for "Not applicable" or "Not observed." Use it when appropriate. Not doing so will undermine the rest of the evaluation.
- *Only write what you have reviewed during feedback.* In almost all circumstances, the learner should not read something for the first time in an evaluation. As described previously, learners

will become angry to see something in their evaluation that was not communicated to them during the time you worked with them. They will feel frustrated that they were not given the opportunity to work on the area needing improvement. It is unwise to evaluate someone in an area about which he or she was not even aware that he or she was doing poorly.

- *If there is a rating scale, use the anchors.* There is tremendous grade inflation in medical education, and many evaluators restrict their ratings to the highest number on the scale. If behavioral anchors are present (i.e., examples of what a number means) read the anchors and use them when making ratings. Think critically about each item you are asked to evaluate, and try to differentiate performance in each of the different competencies. Try to rate each individual or particular skill rather than circling the same rating across all competencies.

- *If there is space for open-ended comments, make them specific.* Many assessment forms include spaces for open-ended comments. Useful comments are those that are specific, that describe relevant competencies and highlight strengths and weaknesses, providing specific examples of both. You need to know what competencies the course director is interested in so that your comments address relevant and important areas. Again, knowledge of the performance standard is needed for comments to be most useful, because comments can than identify objectively where the trainee is compared with the expectation of where he or she should be.

- *Complete your evaluations in a timely manner.* There are several reasons why timely completion of evaluations is important. First, it can be difficult to provide a specific evaluation if months lapse between when you worked with a learner and when you complete the evaluation. Second, learners might contest the accuracy of your evaluation if it is completed months after a course or a rotation. Third, accrediting bodies (i.e., the LCME) often set standards for when students must receive evaluations or course grades. Waiting too long to complete evaluations could therefore jeopardize the school's accreditation status.

Words to the Wise
- Set goals and objectives with your learner. This is the foundation of feedback. Think of it as "feed-up." Where is the learner going?
- Increase the amount of direct observation that you do, because this is the focus of your feedback. Talk with a colleague about feasible strategies for increasing the amount of direct observation you do.
- Seek the learner's self-assessment before you give feedback. Really listen and respond to what the learner has to say.
- Include positive (reinforcing) and negative (constructive) feedback that is specific, objective, timely, and prioritized. It should answer the question, "What progress is being made toward the goal?"
- Make sure that your feedback has an action plan. Your feedback should "feed-forward" and answer the question "What activities need to be undertaken to make progress?" or "Where to next?"
- Role-play with a mentor or a colleague to practice difficult feedback.
- Consider participating in a workshop about teaching skills or providing feedback to practice your skills.

Ask Your Mentor or Colleagues
- What types of feedback have been challenging for you to give? What made them challenging?
- What strategies have you used to give challenging feedback?
- Was there a time you did not give a trainee feedback and wish you had? Why do you think that happened? How could you prevent it from happening again?

Further Reading

Archer JC. State of the science in health professional education: effective feedback. Med Educ. 2010;44: 101–8.

Branch Jr WT, Paranjape A. Feedback and reflection: teaching methods for clinical settings. Acad Med. 2002;77:1185–8.

Cantillon P, Sargeant J. Giving feedback in clinical settings. BMJ. 2008;337: 1292–4.

Ende J. Feedback in clinical medical education. JAMA. 1983;250:777–81.

Hattie J, Timperley H. The power of feedback. Rev Educ Res. 2007;77: 81–112.

Mann K, van der Vleuten C, Eva K, et al. Tensions in informed self-assessment: how the desire for feedback and reticence to collect and use it can conflict. Acad Med. 2011;86:1120–7.

Mazor KM, Holtman MC, Shchukin Y, Mee J, Katsufrakis PJ. The relationship between direct observation, knowledge, and feedback: results of a national survey. Acad Med. 2011;86(10):S63–8.

Menachery EP, Knight AM, Kolodner K, Wright SM. Physician characteristics associated with proficiency in feedback skills. J Gen Intern Med. 2006;21:440–6.

Milan FB, Parish SJ, Reichgott MJ. A model for educational feedback based on clinical communication skills strategies: beyond the "feedback sandwich". Teach Learn Med. 2006;18(1):42–7.

Van de Ridder JMM, Stokking KM, McGaghie WC, ten Cate OTJ. What is feedback in clinical education? Med Educ. 2008;42:189–97.

How to Approach Mentorship as a Mentee

Amy Becker and Joel Yager

Mentee self-awareness and a thoughtfully conceived professional development plan are crucial to the initiation of successful mentoring partnerships. Also essential is the ability to identify and effectively engage mentors who possess the talents, expertise, and professional connections likely to benefit the mentee.

From the very beginning of the relationship, careful consideration should be given to the structure of mentoring encounters and to expectations for the mentorship experience. Mutually beneficial relationships will best sustain as the result of thorough preparation for meetings, continuous hard work, and ongoing assessment of outcomes.

Termination of mentorships should be an anticipated aspect of relationship progression. Although such terminations may on occasion unfortunately occur as personality conflicts became insurmountable, they most commonly end or fade away in more developmentally appropriate fashion as goals are met or mentees advance to positions of increased autonomy.

Mentorship relationships are dynamic and reciprocal processes. These processes are best guided by the mentee's self-determined goals and career visions that evolve and mature through the interactive and iterative experiences of mentorship.

Department of Psychiatry and Behavioral Sciences, Children's Hospital Colorado, Anschutz Medical Campus, Aurora, CO, USA
e-mail: amy.becker@childrenscolorado.org

© Springer International Publishing Switzerland 2016
L.W. Roberts (ed.), *The Clinician Educator Guidebook*,
DOI 10.1007/978-3-319-27980-0_10

Early- and middle-career physicians, scientists, and clinicians have multiple demands placed on their time, especially within the context of academic medicine. The learning curve is very steep as one takes the developmental step from trainee to faculty. As new faculty are called upon to prioritize their time and rapidly assimilate to the academic culture, it becomes extremely important to utilize time wisely and draw upon available resources to promote an efficient and successful transition.

The relationship between mentor and mentee may be something already familiar to early-career faculty, as the fortunate may have either formally or more serendipitously been matched with an experienced faculty mentor as a student. However, as some studies show that mentorship occurs for only one-half to one-third of faculty members, this is frequently not the case [1].

The concept of mentor dates back to the time of Homer's Odyssey, where we find the goddess Athena disguised as Mentor. Mentor provides guidance and wisdom to Telemachus, as he sets out to find his father Odysseus following victory in the Trojan War. More contemporary literature and research carries forward a similar view of mentor within the context of business management and medicine. However, a generally accepted operational definition is lacking. In an effort to standardize the construct of mentorship within academia, an Ad Hoc Faculty Mentorship Committee at Johns Hopkins University proposed the following characterization:

> A mentoring relationship is one that may vary along a continuum from informal/short term to formal/long term in which faculty with useful experience, knowledge, skills and wisdom offers advice, information, guidance, support or opportunity to another faculty member or student for that individual's professional development. [2]

Equally as essential as the contribution of the mentor to the relationship are the roles and responsibilities of the mentee. The mentorship relationship is a dynamic relationship, one that is mutually beneficial and inclusive of both personal and professional gains. This relationship has been identified as influential in the decision of trainees and early-career faculty to enter and remain in academic medicine. Its numerous potential benefits include, but are not limited to, increased self-confidence, improved overall career satisfaction, greater productivity, and an improved sense of professional community [3, 4]. As mentorship affects quality of life and professional choices during formative career-building years, mentees must empower themselves with knowledge about how to create and sustain successful mentoring relationships.

How to Get Started

Self-Assessment

Starting with the fundamental belief that mentees are ultimately responsible for their own professional growth and development, an honest self-assessment is the first step in determining readiness and goodness of fit with any potential mentor. Borrowing once again from our Greek ancestors, Socrates urges us to "know thyself." The initiation of the mentorship relationship is mediated by the personality style of the mentee. Management research has shown that individuals with an internal locus of control, emotional stability, and high self-monitoring experience greater success [5]. Interpersonal effectiveness and well-developed social skills are additionally important assets, as they promote successful networking and self-promotion. Mentees should consider their own personal styles, identify which traits will lend themselves to successful initiation, and capitalize on their assets. These and other elements that mentees should consider and monitor in the course of preparing for, initiating, and sustaining mentorship relationships are listed in Table 10.1.

As personal qualities are being considered, thinking should additionally be expanded to include consideration of values and priorities, particularly those that are considered a requisite part of any successful relationship. Honesty, trust, and integrity are important traits to consider, as a relationship with a mentor will require a certain amount of self-disclosure and receipt of critical feedback. There is also often a power differential within a mentoring relationship and likely collaboration on scholarly work, which further elevates the need for mutual respect and collegiality.

Moving beyond character and values, it is important for mentees to consider any personal preferences they may have when selecting a mentor. Trainees and early-career faculty may prefer to

Table 10.1 Mentee checklist

Before contacting potential mentors

1. Personal reflection on character and values

2. Mentor preferences

3. Self-assessment of strengths and weaknesses
   - (a) Personal
     - Skills
       - Strengths
       - Weaknesses
     - Knowledge
       - Strengths
       - Weaknesses
   - (b) Professional
     - Skills
       - Strengths
       - Weaknesses
     - Knowledge
       - Strengths
       - Weaknesses

4. Professional and personal development plans and aspirations
   - (a) 3-month goals
     - Clinical
     - Teaching
     - Research
     - Personal/family
   - (b) 1-year goals
     - Clinical
     - Teaching
     - Research
     - Personal/family
   - (c) 5-year goals
     - Clinical
     - Teaching
     - Research
     - Personal/family

5. Identify prospective mentors
   - (a) Type (s) of mentorship
   - (b) Local contacts
   - (c) Regional and national contacts

(continued)

Table 10.1 (continued)

Before contacting potential mentors
Initiating contact with potential mentors
(a) Write letter of intent
(b) Update and send curriculum vitae
(c) Schedule meeting
Maintaining and sustaining mentorships
(a) Contact log
(b) Review and update CV
(c) Review specific elements of professional development plan
(d) Review work in progress (grant applications, manuscripts, project proposals, curriculum projects, productivity measures, etc.)

work with a mentor of the same gender or race, as it may enhance the sense of identification and understanding. It may be additionally important to explore the importance of the location of the mentor. While long-distance mentoring may have the advantage of accessing skills or knowledge that are not available to mentees at their home institution, Allen et al. found that mentees perceived more successful career mentoring from mentors within same department, as location impacted availability and interaction frequency, which subsequently enriched the relationship [6].

The next step in a comprehensive self-assessment is to inventory skill and knowledge strengths and weaknesses within both personal and professional domains. Starting with the personal domain, mentees should reflect upon such capabilities as stress management and maintenance of the work–life balance. Professionally, mentees should consider all facets of their career development, including clinical, teaching, and research and begin to focus their energies on the pursuit of excellence in their areas of interest. What naturally follows will be drafting a professional development plan, which includes short-term, mid-range, and long-term goals. A professional development plan should outline the plan for growth in the specific areas of interest and will not only allow mentees to begin to visualize the roadmap to the success that they seek but enable mentees to identify the specific expertise they try to find in a mentor and to make selections based on their individual needs.

Mentor Assessment

Once a mentee's self-assessment is completed and clarity is achieved about specific needs, the next step is to identify mentorship that will best meet those requirements. Formal mentoring programs exist at some institutions, and by utilizing processes already in place, mentees will have an easier time gathering information and making initial connections. In the absence of a formal process, mentees should be proactive in outreach to peers and senior faculty. Identifying faculty with similar interests and complementary talents is crucial, but equally important is determining interest and availability for mentoring. Mentees should ascertain whether potential mentors have reputations for successful mentoring, which will reflect their enthusiasm, abilities, and commitment to the process. It is also important for mentees to align themselves with senior faculty who are accomplished and established within their areas of expertise, as they are most likely to have both theoretical and practical "know-how" and the ability to promote professional networking.

Mentees should appreciate that there are various forms of mentoring, including dyadic, group mentoring, peer mentoring, and mosaic mentoring. Dyadic mentoring describes the more traditional form of mentoring, the one-on-one relationship with a more senior and experienced counterpart. Individual mentors may be called upon for overall guidance and support with life and career planning, but they may also be selected for guidance in areas of specific competency building, such as technical or administrative capacities. Group mentoring may also include the influence and presence of an experienced faculty member; however, in these cases, the experienced individual is providing wisdom and guidance to a group of early-career faculty, often as a way to extend the expertise of a limited resource. Peer mentoring can also take the form of group mentoring, but without the immediate availability of senior influence or input. Peer mentoring can be beneficial by creating an environment of support and problem solving for individuals at the same developmental level. Models for peer mentoring groups have been described, one such group at Duke University, which heralds over 4 years of member retention and measured results such as numerous publications, national presentations, and successful competition for career development awards [7]. Finally, mentees may consider mosaic mentoring, essentially a combination of all forms of mentorship. Seldom does one individual have the ability to meet all of the complex and evolving needs of the mentee, so enlisting the support and guidance of multiple individuals will often yield the best results.

Next Steps

Engagement

Once the prospective mentor or mentors have been identified by the mentee, the next step will be to initiate contact. The initial contact may be in the form of an email or telephone call, to briefly explain the purpose of the outreach, to establish the availability and potential interest of the mentor, and to schedule a meeting. Depending on circumstances, the mentee should also consider sending a curriculum vitae (CV) and cover letter of intent to any prospective mentor prior to a personal meeting, approaching the relationship much as one would with any potential employer. Providing information in advance will not only allow the mentors to gauge if they can meet the mentee's specific needs but will also allow them to consider whether they have time and interest to invest in the commitment. In some instances, mentees will have to be persistent, since not all requests are going to be met with quick acceptance. Mentees may also discover that while someone may appear in theory to be an ideal match by reputation and credentials, a personal meeting may rapidly uncover incompatibilities in personalities.

At the time of the initial meeting, mentees should be clear about their requests and highlight what they have to offer the relationship in time, energy, and talents. Mentees are well served by following up the initial meeting with a written summary of the discussions and, regardless of outcome, expressing appreciation for the opportunity to have met. If the potential mentor turns out not to be a good match, the mentee should consider asking that person for additional personal recommendations, based on their understanding of the mentee's needs and approach to the mentoring relationship. While they may not be suited to meet the needs the mentee has identified at the outset of initial contact, senior faculty may still serve as resources and be able to make connections within one's professional community.

Maintenance

Once a mentor relationship or mentorship team is established, the mentee should utilize the first few meetings to solidify the agenda for the relationship, for example, determining the frequency of visits, typically every 2–4 weeks, and agreed upon goals. In advance of these meetings, mentees should always do their homework, demonstrating their commitment to the relationship by coming to mentorship meetings well prepared.

Communication will be always be important and may become increasingly nuanced as mentees become better acquainted with their mentors, particularly as challenges begin to arise. Mentees are well served by being mindful of the workplace, setting realistic expectations for oneself and for the mentors, accepting feedback gracefully, and being active listeners who are inviting of and open to constructive critique. The challenge for mentees is to find optimal balance between unconditionally accepting and questioning the voice of experience, being open to growth and change while maintaining one's own personal identity and career goals.

Mentees must also remain vigilant about maintaining professional and personal boundaries, since mentorship relationships are inevitably based on an imbalance of power in the relationship. They need to guard against being exploited by a mentor for personal or professional gain and to be aware of becoming too dependent upon these relationships. Developing an overidealizing view of the mentor may potentially compromise the mentee's ability to develop independent thought and ideas [5]. The ideal mentor can altruistically separate his or her own personal agenda from the agenda of the mentee and enhance and support the mentee's ability to see an expanded vision for their future.

Outcomes

Measuring the outcomes—and, hopefully, successes—of any mentoring relationship has both subjective and objective aspects and starts with the assessments of the participating mentee and mentor utilizing the mutually agreed upon goals and professional development plan as benchmarks. Updating and reviewing the mentee's evolving CV and academic products, both in progress and as they are completed, will serve as helpful measures of progress and aid in the systematic assessment of professional development across all dimensions. More formally structured tools for institutional or mentee oversight have been created that track specific areas of individual and programmatic interest [8, 9]. Business and psychology literature has also informed academic physicians concerned with fostering successful careers. Both intrinsic and extrinsic factors such as financial remuneration, promotion, grants, publications, clinical achievement, administrative achievement, and life satisfaction are all included in these considerations. These models may offer helpful suggestions for early-career faculty members attempting to create their own all inclusive visions for success [10].

Termination

Recognizing when a relationship with a mentor has run its course can be challenging. Relationships can electively be terminated prior to meeting objectives, as personality or professional conflicts become insurmountable obstacles to progress. Relationships may additionally end as professional appointments change, making the necessary time commitment unmanageable or location incompatible with frequent meetings. Relationships with mentors also approach termination as goals are met and mentees progress to positions of increased autonomy. As is developmentally appropriate, the mentor role may evolve to that of colleague and/or friend, and the mentee may in turn move into the role of mentor to other faculty members, thereby transmitting the legacy of mentorship to the next generation of aspiring physicians, clinicians, and scientists.

Conclusion

Mentorship relationships, seemingly part of the human condition, have undoubtedly been around since eons of time prior to the eighth century BC—the time of Mentor and Telemachus. The numerous benefits of these relationships result from hard work and commitment to the process. Early-career faculty are advised to educate themselves as to how to make the most of their mentorship experiences. These dynamic and reciprocal processes should be guided primarily by the mentee's self-determined goals and career vision that evolve and mature through the processes of mentorship.

Words to the Wise
- Since effective mentoring is likely to enrich and positively impact professional development and career accomplishments, up and coming academic faculty members should energetically pursue mentorship early in their careers.
- Although ideal matches may not come immediately or easily, mentees should proactively and persistently pursue mentorship. The good matches ultimately achieved are well worth the effort.
- In order to best maximize the benefits of these relationships, mentees should commit themselves by thorough preparation for meetings with mentors and diligence in following them up by attending to action items and assigned goals.

Ask Your Mentor or Colleagues
- What are your interests and experiences in mentoring early-career faculty members?
- What are your areas of interest and expertise?
- What is your availability for mentor ship?
- What are your expectations of your mentee and/or yourself as a mentor in this relationship?

References

1. Carey EC, Weissman DE. Understanding and finding mentorship: a review for junior faculty. J Palliat Med. 2010;13:1373–9.
2. Berk RA, Mortimer R, Walton-Moss B, Yeo TP. Measuring the effectiveness of faculty mentoring relationships. Acad Med. 2005;80(1):66–71.
3. Sambunjak D, Straus S, Marusic A. Mentoring in academic medicine: a systematic review. JAMA. 2006;296(9):1103–15.
4. Palepu A, Friedman RH, Barnett RC, et al. Junior faculty members' mentoring relationships and their professional development in US medical schools. Acad Med. 1998;73(3):318–23.
5. Rodenhauser P, Rudisill JR, Dvorak R. Skills for mentors and proteges applicable to psychiatry. Acad Med. 2000;24(1):14–27.
6. Allen TD, Eby LT, Lentz E. Mentorship behaviors and mentorship quality associated with formal mentoring programs: closing the gap between research and practice. J Appl Psychol. 2006;91(3):567–78.
7. Johnson KS, Hastings SN, Purser JL, Whitson H. The junior faculty laboratory: an innovative model of peer mentoring. Acad Med. 2011;86(12):1577–82.
8. Waitzkin H, Yager J, Parker T, Duran B. Mentoring partnerships for minority faculty and graduate students in mental health services research. Acad Psychiatry. 2006;30(3):205–17.
9. Keyser DJ, Lakoski JM, Lara-Cinisomo S, et al. Advancing institutional efforts to support research mentorship: a conceptual framework and self-assessment tool. Acad Med. 2008;83(3):217–25.
10. Rubio DM, Primack BA, Switzer GE, et al. A comprehensive career-success model for physician–scientists. Acad Med. 2011;86(12):1571–6.

How to Write a Case Report

11

Richard Balon and Eugene Beresin

As Borus [1] pointed out, writing for publication has been an "essential component of a successful career in academic medicine." Writing and publishing a case report may be, and frequently is, a starting point of writing for publication. On the other hand, as Martyn [2] mentions, case reports are at the bottom of scientific writing and at the bottom of what counts as reliable evidence for clinical decision-making. Thus, one may ask, why start writing with a case report? There are various valid reasons. Most beginning faculty members are not involved in conducting studies and writing up their results. Case reports may offer a better and quicker start in writing than an original observation or a review. Writing a case report could be a very good starting point of the process of learning how to write for publication. Last, but not least, case reports provide interesting clinical and educational information to the field of medicine. Martyn [2] mentioned a couple of classic case reports that alerted other physicians to start further investigations of far-reaching significance. And, as Roselli and Otero stated, "The case report is far from dead," in 2001 MEDLINE crossed the

R. Balon, M.D. (✉)
Departments of Psychiatry and Behavioral Neurosciences and
Anesthesiology, Wayne State University School of Medicine, Detroit,
MI, USA
e-mail: rbalon@wayne.edu

© Springer International Publishing Switzerland 2016
L.W. Roberts (ed.), *The Clinician Educator Guidebook*,
DOI 10.1007/978-3-319-27980-0_11

barrier of 1,000,000 case reports, and 40,000 new cases enter MEDLINE each year [3].

This chapter provides a guide on how to write a case report for publication on the basis of available articles and our own experience.

Types of Case Reports

There are various categories or types of case reports. The two main types are the regular, clinically oriented case report, published in a full case report format (see below) or as a letter to the editor; and the educational case report, which includes a broader description, discussion by an expert or multiple experts, and also possibly continuing medical education material (e.g., questions). Some journals use case reports as a medium for continuing medical education [4].

Green and Johnson [4] outlined three types of case reports that tend to be published: (a) diagnostic or assessment reports, (b) treatment or management reports, and (c) educational reports. According to Iles and Piepho [5], most of the case reports fall into one of the following categories: "(1) an unexpected association between two relatively uncommon diseases or symptoms, (2) an unexpected event or outcome in the course of observing or treating a patient, (3) findings that shed new light on the possible pathogenesis of a disease or an adverse drug effect, (4) unique or rare features of a disease, or (5) unique therapeutic approaches." Similarly, Wright and Kouroukis [6] distinguish four kinds of case reports: "(a) the unique case that appears to represent a newly described syndrome or disease, (b) the case with an unexpected association of two diseases that may represent a causal relation, (c) the "outlier" case representing a variation from the expected pattern, and (d) the case with a surprising evolution that suggests a therapeutic or adverse drug effect." Both Iles and Piepho [5] and Wright and Kouroukis [6] draw from Huth's book on writing and publishing in medicine (see the recommended reading list at the end of this chapter).

How to Decide Whether, When, and Why to Write a Case Report

Writing just for the sake of writing should not be the reason for writing anything. The decision to write a case report should be based on the fact that this case report is going to provide new and useful knowledge to the field, unless the author is asked to prepare an educational case report. Thus, prospective authors "should resist the urge to report a case that announces a finding that, although new, makes no difference in understanding a disease or improving therapy" [5]. Green and Johnson [4] summarized the literature on reasons for submitting a case report for publication: (1) to present an unusual or unknown disorder; (2) to present unusual etiology for a case; (3) to present a challenging differential diagnosis; (4) to describe mistakes in health care, their causes and consequences; (5) to describe an unusual setting for care; (6) to present information that cannot be reproduced due to ethical reasons; (7) to illustrate a clinical hypothesis; (8) to prompt a new hypothesis; (9) to disconfirm a hypothesis; (10) to support a hypothesis; (11) to stimulate further research; (12) to make an original contribution to the literature; (13) to offer new insight into the pathogenesis of disease; (14) to describe unusual or puzzling clinical features; (15) to describe improved or unique technical procedures; (16) to describe the historical development of a field or movement; (17) to report unusual drug–drug, drug–food, or drug–nutrient interactions; (18) to describe rare or novel adverse reactions to care; and (19) to study the mechanism of a disease. While this list seems exhaustive, it is not (further reasons include, e.g., a novel treatment approach), yet it certainly provides enough guidance.

A clinically-oriented educational case report should follow the specific requirements of each particular journal (e.g., the New England Journal of Medicine, the American Journal of Psychiatry) and its editorial leadership.

A purely educational case report usually describes a new teaching method or approach or ethical issues in teaching. It may be published in a format of a special column (e.g., Educational Resource Column in *Academic Psychiatry*).

What to Do Before Starting to Write a Case Report

Having an interesting, challenging, or unusual case does not necessarily mean that one will be successful in publishing it. Writing a case report, like any other writing for publication, requires a considerable amount of thinking it through and preparation. Wright and Kouroukis [6] provide some advice on what to do prior to writing a case report to improve the chances that it will be published. They start with the well-known adage, "read, read, and read some more." One has to be familiar with the literature to know whether one's case is really as unique, interesting, or useful as one thinks. In the beginning, the author has to conduct a solid literature review (PubMed, MEDLINE, or other search systems) to see whether similar or related cases have been published in the past. Wright and Kouroukis [6] suggest that one does a search beyond just the disease/condition/medication and adds a search that includes the word "case report" across a large database. The literature search will confirm or disconfirm whether one's case report is unique or interesting. However, a previously published case report of a disease, symptom, or side effect does not necessarily mean that one's case is not publishable. The case report at hand needs to be assessed for unique aspects in comparison to previously published ones. Our general knowledge may also benefit from the addition of a rare or unique case to a previously published case report. Such a case may suggest that the presumably rare or extremely rare condition, situation, or event is not as rare as previously thought and should be studied further. Careful reading of previously published case reports and literature about the disease or treatment in general may also help in preparation of one's manuscript.

When considering one's case report for publication, one should also be aware of the fact that some case reports or case series may have far-reaching and not always positive implications. Procopio [7] warns us that "the publication of a one-off case report of an adverse effect can profoundly influence clinical practice on the basis of a freak event," while "the cases of the hundreds of thousands of people who have been safely and successfully treated with these medications are not published because no one wants to state the obvious." This statement outlines the scope of responsibility one has when deciding whether or not to publish a singular finding. Hence, there is a professional duty tied to the publication of a case report.

In addition to a lot of preparatory reading, Wright and Kouroukis [6] recommend that one orders the appropriate tests to confirm the diagnosis; obtain informed consent (also for additional tests; for further discussion, see below); maintain patient confidentiality (examples include deleting patient's initials, avoiding identifying details unless essential, and masking crucial parts of the patient's photograph); involve consultants early; request an autopsy if indicated; save blood samples if indicated; and discuss the case report with the editorial staff of the journal to which one intends to submit the case report. These suggestions apply to both retrospective (a description of something that already happened, e.g., symptom, diagnosis, side effect) and prospective case reports (e.g., planned attempt to treat a condition with an approved medication that has not been used in this indication but may intuitively make sense or patient reports that an accidental use of a medication helped him or her and the clinician wants to verify it).

The preparation of a prospective case report may slightly differ from the usual descriptive, retrospective case report. One may consider using various measures, such as rating scales or serial laboratory testing. Again, reading about the condition and/or treatment beforehand applies. Prospective case reports or case series may require approval of the Ethics Committee or Institutional Review Board (IRB) prior to starting any intervention (observational cases may be exempt from IRB approval—one should always inquire at one's local institution).

Choice of a Journal and Journal Rules/ Requirements

We discuss the choice of the journal where one would like to submit a case report as it may be a crucial decision with regard to getting the manuscript published. There are journals that, as a matter of editorial policy, do not publish case reports, either because they do not consider their scientific value to be significant or because of space considerations. Some journals that do publish case reports as of this writing include the American Journal of

Psychiatry (as a letter to the editor or invited educational case), American Journal of Psychotherapy, Annals of Clinical Psychiatry, British Journal of Psychiatry (mostly as a letter to the editor), Canadian Journal of Psychiatry, General Hospital Psychiatry (full-fledged cases), Journal of Clinical Psychiatry (both as a full-fledged case report and as a letter to the editor), JAMA (as a letter to the editor), Journal of Clinical Psychopharmacology, Psychopathology (full-fledged cases), Psychosomatics, Psychotherapy and Psychosomatics (as a letter to the editor), New England Journal of Medicine (Clinical Cases), and Harvard Review of Psychiatry (Clinical Challenges).

One also needs to make sure that the case report reaches the proper audience [8] and thus needs to select an appropriate journal (e.g., a psychotherapy journal does not provide the most appropriate audience for a case report describing a side effect of a new medication) and tailor the manuscript to a specific audience. Reviewing the contents of the journal during the past year or 2 may be helpful to see whether the case report would appeal to the editor and the readership of the selected journal.

The authors should also consult the Information for Authors of the selected journal to make sure that their manuscript conforms to the policies of the journal as to the format, scope, number of words, illustrations, number and format of references, and the method of submission. At the present time, almost all journals accept manuscripts via the internet and electronic manuscript processing systems (e.g., Manuscript Central). The journal instructions inform mostly on style (i.e., word limitation, pages, figures or illustrations, tables, references, need for an abstract, key words, and consent form) [9]. Journals usually do not provide much information on the contents of case reports. According to one study [8], 60 % of journals publishing case reports provided information on whether the case had to be unusual, 55 % whether an instructive or teaching point was required, 26 % whether the case should be original and innovative, and 6 % of journals considered hypothesis generation a reason for reporting the case. Only a small portion of journals requiring informed consent actually provided a consent form. The amount of advice for authors is usually fairly limited. It might be informative to read recent cases in the journal to appreciate the style, format, or other details and to review the clinical material for preparation with a senior academic psychiatrist and/or the hospital's general counsel regarding the necessity for informed consent. In addition, many editors are happy to answer specific questions an author might have regarding preparation of a manuscript.

Special attention should be paid to the word number limitations or the expected length of a case report. The manuscript may be rejected merely on the basis of violating this requirement. Many journals, especially those publishing case reports as a letter to the editor only, allow no more than 500 words. According to the study by Sorinola et al. [9], the recommended length of case reports in various journals varied from 500 to 2000 words with a median of 1000 words. Educational case reports of some major journals and case reports in some psychoanalytical journals allow for a larger number of words. In any case, authors may check with the editorial office of the particular journal if they feel that the case report cannot be summarized within the word limit specified by the journal.

Informed Consent and Confidentiality/ Patient Privacy

Patient privacy has to be preserved. The patient cannot be identified from the case description or any other fact published in the case report. To address the issues of confidentiality and privacy, the International Committee of Medical Journal Editors (mostly major medical journals and the National Library of Medicine) published a statement in 1995 regarding patients' rights to privacy in published case reports [10]. According to this statement, "Patients have rights to privacy that should not be infringed without informed consent. Identifying information should not be published in written descriptions, photographs, or pedigrees unless the information is essential for scientific purposes and the patient (or parent or guardian) gives written informed consent for publication. Informed consent for this purpose requires that the patient be shown the manuscript to be published. Identifying details should be omitted if they are not essential, but patient data should never be altered or falsified in an attempt to attain anonymity. Complete anonymity is difficult to achieve, and informed consent should be obtained if there is any doubt. For example, masking of the eye region in photographs is inadequate protection" [10]. Singer [11] described some exceptions to this guideline, such as when the patient is long deceased and has no living relatives, the interaction with the patient was long ago (approximately 15 years), all extraneous information that might help identification is excluded, and even if the patient were to identify himself or herself, the described events are unlikely to cause offense. (Singer's article [11] includes the British Medical Journal's detailed policy on consent to the publication of patient information.) The circumstances of obtaining an informed consent in psychiatry and especially the area of psychotherapy could be a bit more complicated, as Levine and Stagno [12] pointed out. They suggested that in some situations, requesting informed consent may be unethical, can harm patients, and may erode the use of case reports as a valuable teaching method in psychiatry and psychotherapy. When in doubt, it is always useful to consult a senior academic psychiatrist with expertise in psychotherapy.

The identifying information should clearly be omitted, and using actual patient names or initials is prohibited (e.g., one can write either "A 35-year-old male" or "Mr. A. was a 35-year-old male" instead). Most of the journals have not historically required the patient's consent to publish the case in well-anonymized case reports. However, as Green and Johnson [4] pointed out, "Case reports tend to report on unusual situations and patient identity may be compromised because of the unique qualities of the case." Thus, more recently, some journals started to require that the author(s) submit a specific consent form signed by the patient. This specific form may be obtained from the particular journal, and author(s) should check with the editorial office whether a written patient consent is required and under what conditions it could be omitted.

Whether or not to get an informed consent from a patient is not a clear-cut issue. Nevertheless, we believe that in properly anonymized retrospective cases, informed consent for publication is not needed. Prospective cases or case series may not only require an informed consent but also an approval from the local institutional review board (the prospective author should always check his or her institutional policies).

Authorship

The situation of a single-author case report or any article is simple. Anything involving more than one author could become complicated. As a general rule, only persons involved in preparing and/ or writing the manuscript should be included as authors of the manuscript. The extent of involvement may vary but generally should include the acquisition, analysis, and discussion of the data (here of the case report), reviewing the literature, drafting and/or reviewing/revising the manuscript, and approving the final form of the manuscript prior to submission for publication. The person who has done the most work should be the first author, and the order of the rest of the authors should be determined by the amount of contribution. In many published studies the last author is usually the senior author, leader of the research group, or chair (in all cases, hopefully, involved in preparation and/or editing of the manuscript). Case reports are frequently generated by early-career faculty members or residents/fellows who may not be the attending physicians of the patient described in the case report. In those cases, the attending physician could/should become the senior, last author, again, only if his or her contribution to the case report was substantial, as outlined before. We recommend that the order of authorship is discussed and agreed upon prior to starting the work on the manuscript. The person who has done the most work does not want to be in a situation in which he or she is told by a senior colleague after all the work is done, "Since this was my patient, I will be the first author."

Many publications include a long list of authors. This may, especially for a short, concise, simple case report, raise questions about the involvement of all authors. As Har-El [13] aptly asked, "Does it take a village to write a case report?" Clearly not. Some authors may obviously be what is called "honorary authors" who are bequeathed by "gift authorship." Many of these honorary authors are chairs or senior researchers. Early-career authors could understandably feel obliged to include their mentors. Nevertheless, the practice of "gift authorship" raises ethical concerns and should be abandoned. It may be up to the senior authors to reject authorship. An important rule of thumb to consider is whether an individual made any significant contribution to the finished product.

Those who may have contributed to the case report preparation to a lesser extent than that of an author may be acknowledged or thanked in the Acknowledgements section of the case report.

Organization/Components of the Case Report

A case report, like any other manuscript, should have a certain structure. The lower the number of words allowed, the simpler the case report structure. Shorter case reports should include the following elements: Title/Title page; Introduction; Case description; Discussion/Conclusion; References; Acknowledgements; and if required by the journal, a statement about possible conflict of interest. Some case reports may not even need an introduction and may go directly to the case description followed by a brief discussion.

Longer or more complicated case reports may consist of a Title/Title page; Abstract; Introduction; Case report—Methods and Results (especially in prospective cases testing a hypothesis or new management approach); Discussion; Conclusion; Acknowledgements; References; and if required, a statement about possible conflict of interest.

Both shorter and more complex case reports may include tables and figures. Some journals may also require identification of key words that will be used for the search after the case report is published (e.g., schizophrenia, antipsychotics). To select key words use general terms from Index Medicus and other databases and also include words unique to the specific case.

Tables and figures should not duplicate the text [8] but, rather, should help to summarize and shorten it.

Title/Title Page

The title should be as brief and succinct as possible [4] and should inform the reader what the topic of the case report is. When "clever or artistic" titles are used, a subtitle should be added so that the reader could more easily determine the focus of the case report [4].

The title page should include, in addition to the title, a listing of the authors, possibly the authors' titles, the authors' affiliations (the primary affiliation is usually sufficient), the name of the corresponding author (usually the first author, unless he or she left the institution or is not involved with managing the case report anymore), and the corresponding author's contact information (address, phone, fax number, e-mail address).

Some journals may not require a title page, and then the author(s)' names and affiliation(s) may be placed at the end of the case report.

Abstract

An abstract is not always a component of the case report. However, if allowed/required, it is a very important part that summarizes the case and the message of the case. The abstract together with the title are entered into computer databases and indexing systems and thus will help those searching through these systems decide whether they would like to retrieve a particular case report [4, 14]. The abstracts are either structured or unstructured, and most journals have a word limit for the abstract. The abstract of a case report would most likely not be structured but narrative.

Introduction

The introduction should state the purpose, subject, value, pertinence, and worthiness of the report [4, 8]. It should include pertinent references—for instance, previously published similar cases or review articles focused on this topic. The writer should remember that the introduction is just that and not an extensive overview of the literature. Thus, like the rest of the manuscript, it should be brief, concise, and straight to the point. The introduction should end with a link connecting it to the case description and discussion to follow [8]. For instance, one may say, "Our case describes a more severe consequences of the sudden withdrawal of medication X than those previously published."

Case Description

The case description should start with a brief patient description, including pertinent demographic data (age, sex, possibly, if salient to the case, ethnicity, marital status, and occupation) followed by a brief history of the illness/disorder/symptoms, pertinent elements of patient history (e.g., developmental issues related to the presented psychopathology; previous response to or tolerability of similar medications; family history of similar symptomatology); abbreviated mental status examination or important present illness symptomatology; and, depending on the specific case, the results of physical examination, diagnostic tests; laboratory tests (include the specific lab's normal values); imaging results; and finally, in treatment/side effect description cases, outcome of the intervention or natural course. As Green and Johnson [4] suggest, the case description should thus "present the most salient parts of the case presentation; focus on the primary aspects of the patient's condition and the main outcome measures used to track patient progress prior to delivering care; briefly describe methods used to care for the patient and/or assess the patient's status; and briefly summarize outcomes of care, including changes in the primary outcome measures."

DeBakey and DeBakey [8] suggest that one should follow the ABCs in writing a case description and the rest of the case report: Keep it *a*ccurate, *b*rief and *c*lear. One should avoid the liturgy of daily symptomatology or results and select only the pertinent facts.

Discussion

The discussion is the most important part of the case report [14]. It should put the case into a broader perspective, pointing out the uniqueness, its relationship to other published cases (similarities, differences), and summarizing how the case contributes to the literature [4] using relevant references. The discussion should present a justification for publishing this case report. The author should also anticipate and discuss any alternative explanations [8] and be aware that the patient has possibly withheld some important explanation that may provide an alternative explanation [8]. The limitations of the case and its explanation should also be included. The discussion should end with a conclusion/summary—"the take-home message." The reader should learn a piece of pertinent clinical information. The conclusion may also include some recommendations—either for further study or for modification of clinical care based on the outcome of this case. However, one should avoid sweeping generalizations, unwarranted speculations [8], and vague recommendations. Writing just that "more research is needed" is inadequate [4].

Squires [15] provides examples of questions authors should contemplate when writing the discussion/comments: Is the evidence to support the diagnosis presented adequately? Is the evidence to present the author's recommendation presented adequately? Are other plausible explanations considered and refuted? Are the implications and relevance of the case discussed? Do the authors indicate directions for future investigations or management of similar cases?

Acknowledgements

A note at the end of the report should acknowledge colleagues who assisted with the work yet did not fulfill the authorship criteria [4] and support staff who helped with writing, editing, and proofreading the manuscript. Broad gratitude to numerous senior people or family members for their support should be avoided.

References

Most journals that publish case reports specify the number of references allowed (usually 10–15, but more references may be allowed if pertinent to the case). The references used should be from peer-reviewed journals, unless it is absolutely necessary to use other sources. The references should be relevant, pertinent to the case; the author should not be over-inclusive to demonstrate his or her scholarship. A single reference may be enough [4].

Most journals specify the format of references, and thus the author should carefully check the instructions for the authors for this specification.

One caveat: As DeBakey and DeBakey [8] caution, one should never transfer a reference cited in another article without reading it critically. One should be cautious about citing anything from the abstract, as abstracts frequently do not match the contents exactly or are too vague.

Tables, Figures, Illustrations

Tables, figures, and illustrations can be very useful and can make a case report more interesting and easier to understand. Their inclusion may depend on the journal's rules and specifications. As noted earlier, tables and figures should not duplicate the information provided in the text and vice versa.

We are not discussing here the structure of educational case reports or clinical discussions published in some journals, such as the New England Journal of Medicine or the American Journal of Psychiatry, because these case reports are usually invited by the editor or editorial staff and specifications and requirements are provided. Also, several articles (e.g., refs. [4, 14, 16, 17]) include tables and checklists for a detailed case report structure.

Writing Style

As mentioned, case reports should be accurate, brief, and concise [8], and the language should be vivid. An excellent article by DeBakey and DeBakey [18] exhaustively addresses the issues of style and form. They suggest that the manuscript draft be read and reviewed several times with a focus on accuracy, validity, coherency, grammatical integrity, conciseness and clarity, stylistic grace, rhythm and cadence, and finally for general readability [18]. One should avoid jargon, slang, vogue and vague words, clichés, redundancy, and circumlocution [18]. (The details on language provided by DeBakey and DeBakey [18] are beyond the scope of this chapter, but the interested reader may benefit from this article.) The writing style could also benefit from some suggestions of Resnick and Soliman [19] in their chapter on draftsmanship of forensic reports, such as the following: Multisyllabic words reduce readability and comprehension. Sentences of 20–25 words have the greatest readability. One should use common words (e.g., "after" rather than "subsequent to"). Acronyms should be avoided unless widely known. Needless words should not be used. Pregnant negatives (such as what symptoms are not present) should be avoided. One should be cautious about using haughty, pompous, and absolute ("never," "always") or hedge ("apparently," "supposedly") words.

DeBakey and DeBakey [18] recommend that after the first draft of a case report is done, it is best laid aside for several weeks before beginning a critical revision of the text (before submission). Resnick and Soliman [19] suggest that proofreading out loud or backwards may allow for some overlooked errors to be discovered. Others [16] suggest asking oneself, "Would I have taken the trouble to read this case report if I came across it in a journal? What lessons can be learnt?"

Post-submission (Review Process and Galley Proofs)

Once the case report is submitted (via the Internet in most cases), the period of waiting for the decision starts. After the initial screening, most journals send the manuscript for a peer review by experts in the field (those may be selected from the authors cited in the references). Some journals ask the authors to specify preferred reviewers and reviewers that should preferably not be used.

It may take from several weeks to several months to receive a response from the journal. One should avoid contacting the journal and urging to get a response "as soon as possible." Most journals try to respond in a timely fashion. The authors should also realize that while an outright rejection is possible, an outright acceptance, without revision, is rare. When the journal asks authors to revise and resubmit the manuscript, the editor attaches the comments by the reviewers and, at times, some editorial comments. The comments are usually quite helpful, asking for clarifications, pointing out discrepancies, bringing to the authors' attention other references/sources of information. The authors should answer all reviewers' comments in a positive, constructive, and informative manner. In case of comments or recommendations that could not be answered (e.g., if information is not available), it should be stated that one cannot address this suggestion and the reasons should be explained. The response should be accompanied by a letter to the editor describing all the changes that were made, those suggested by the reviewers and also those the authors may have implemented on their own while rereading the manuscript.

Once the manuscript is accepted, the editorial office informs the authors and forwards the final version of the manuscript to the publisher. The authors are also asked to complete a copyright form transferring the publishing rights/ownership to the journal/publisher. The last pieces of correspondence before publication are the so-called proofs or galley proofs. This is the typeset version of the manuscript, looking usually exactly like it is going to look in the journal. The author(s) are asked to proof the final version for accuracy, language, and so on. As many journals implement editorial changes in the language, we strongly urge authors to review the proofs very carefully. The editorial changes may, at times, change the meaning of the sentences and, in all fairness, the editorial staff may not be aware of all the case report intricacies, terminology, and meaning. One should return the proofs within the specified deadline (usually 24–48 h) to the publisher.

Conclusion

Case reports, an important part of the medical literature, are far from dead [3] and are here to stay. They usually provide important and useful clinical information. They have an educational value. They frequently serve as a stepping stone or writing exercise for beginning writers. Writing a good, publishable case report is a skill and requires following certain rules and guidelines outlined in this chapter. The main rule of writing a good case report that has been vetted as interesting and possibly unique and contributing to the literature is to be accurate, brief, concise, and readable.

Words to the Wise
- Be sure your report reaches the proper audience. Selecting the appropriate journal is crucial.
- Determine whether anonymity is achieved. When in doubt, obtain informed consent and consult your hospital legal counsel, IRB, or Ethics Committee, particularly for psychiatry and psychotherapy case reports.
- Establish the order of authorship and its rationale before preparation of the case report.
- Maintain the "ABCs" of the case report: Keep it Accurate, Brief, and Clear. Remember that the discussion is the most important part of the report, justifying its importance, considering its contribution to the field, and also providing limitations and possible alternative explanations.
- Never transfer a reference from another paper without reading all the references thoroughly and critically.
- Set aside the paper before a careful revision and, after thoroughly revising it, ask, "Would I read, understand, and learn from this case report if I came across it in a journal?"

Ask Your Mentor or Colleagues
- Before preparation of the manuscript, ask about the criteria for and order of authorship. It is always valuable to have an outside senior mentor or trusted colleague provide such advice.
- Before submission of the report to a journal, show the report to your mentor and ask: "Is my completed case report unique, valuable, a contribution to knowledge, and relevant to current and future practice? What might I be missing or neglecting in the manuscript?"
- Have a senior author in academic medicine who is not a coauthor of the paper critically review your writing style. Ask, "Is my writing accurate, valid, coherent, concise, clear, and readable? Would you please provide me specific, detailed feedback as if you were a reviewer for a journal?"

(continued)

(continued)
- When you receive a case report for revision and respond to the reviewers' comments, show your revision to a mentor or colleague and ask, "Did I faithfully, respectfully, and effectively address the comments of the reviewers? Please comment if you see areas of persistent weakness."

References

1. Borus JF. Writing for publication. In: Kay J, Silberman EK, Pessar L, editors. Handbook of psychiatric education and faculty development. Washington, DC: American Psychiatric Press; 1999. p. 57–93.
2. Martyn C. Case reports, case series and systematic reviews. Q J Med. 2002;95:197–8.
3. Roselli D, Otero A. The case report is far from dead. Lancet. 2002;359:84.
4. Green BN, Johnson CD. How to write a case report for publication. J Chiropract Med. 2006;5:72–82.
5. Iles RL, Piepho RW. Presenting and publishing case reports. J Clin Pharmacol. 1996;36:573–9.
6. Wright SM, Kouroukis C. Capturing zebras: what to do with a reportable case. Can Med Assoc J. 2000;163:429–31.
7. Procopio M. Publication of case reports. Br J Psychiatry. 2005;187:91.
8. DeBakey L, DeBakey S. The case report. I. Guidelines for preparation. Int J Cardiol. 1983;4:357–64.
9. Sorinola O, Loufowobi O, Coomarasamy A, Khan KS. Instructions to authors for case reporting are limited: a review of a core journal list. BMC Med Educ. 2004;4:4.
10. International Committee of Medical Journal Editors. Protection of patients' rights to privacy. BMJ. 1995;311:1272.
11. Singer PA. Consent to publication of patient information. BMJ. 2004;329:566–8.
12. Levine SB, Stagno SJ. Informed consent for case reports. The ethical dilemma of right to privacy versus pedagogical freedom. J Psychother Pract Res. 2001;10:193–201.
13. Har-El G. Does it take a village to write a case report? Otoralyng Head Neck Surg. 1999;120:787–8.
14. McCarthy LH, Reilly KEH. How to write a case report. Fam Med. 2000;32:190–5.

15. Squires BP. Case reports: what editors want from authors and peer reviewers. Can Med Assoc J. 1989;141:379–80.
16. Chelvarajah R, Bycroft J. Writing and publishing case reports: to road to success. Acta Neurochir (Wien). 2004;146:313–6.
17. Cohen H. How to write a patient case report. Am J Health Syst Pharm. 2006;63:1888–92.
18. DeBakey L, DeBakey S. The case report. II. Style and form. Int J Cardiol. 1984;6:247–54.
19. Resnik PJ, Soliman S. Draftsmanship. In: Buchanan A, Norco MA, editors. The psychiatric report. Principles and practice of forensic writing. New York, NY: Cambridge University Press; 2011. p. 81–92.

Further Reading

Huth FJ. Writing and publishing in medicine, 3rd ed. Baltimore: Williams & Wilkins; 1999 (previously published as *How to write and publish papers in medical sciences*).

How to Review a Manuscript

12

Thomas W. Heinrich

The peer review process in scientific publications is fundamental to the dissemination of worthy medical knowledge. It accomplishes this through its impact on the publication of quality manuscripts and other forms of media that we rely on to inform our clinical practice, educational mission, scientific research, and practice administration. Peer reviewers play an important role in the determination of which information is appropriate for publication as well as ensuring scientific integrity and ethical veracity in the products which are produced. Reviewers should seek to improve the products under review and educate the author(s) in how to implement this improvement in the submission. Furthermore, they must accomplish this feat in an ethical, collegial, prompt, and consistent manner.

The peer review process is not new. It has existed in various forms since the eighteenth century when the Royal Society of London assigned peers to serve on the "Committee on Papers" [1]. This committee's members were to review manuscripts submitted for publication in the Society's journal *Transactions*. This was followed by a relatively informal process in which some

T.W. Heinrich, M.D., F.A.P.M. (✉)
Department of Psychiatry and Behavioral Medicine,
Medical College of Wisconsin, 8701 Watertown Plank Road,
Milwaukee, WI, USA
e-mail: theinric@mcw.edu

© Springer International Publishing Switzerland 2016   169
L.W. Roberts (ed.), *The Clinician Educator Guidebook*,
DOI 10.1007/978-3-319-27980-0_12

editors of journals would seek review of certain articles on a case-by-case basis. It was not until the twentieth century that editors began to formalize the process in which journals used peer reviewers. Editors began to become more reliant on peer reviewers' objective expert advice on helping to determine the appropriateness of the science, significance of the message, and overall quality of the manuscripts submitted for publication in their journals. Today the peer review process has become institutionalized in medical science. It is considered one of the best methods that journals have in selecting appropriate manuscripts for publication and dissemination [2].

Unfortunately the procedure of how one reviews a manuscript is rarely part of the curriculum taught during medical school, residency, or fellowship training. Reviewing is all too often a skill developed in relative isolation early in a physician's academic career with little in the way of feedback or quality assurance. As a result, early-career faculty may find it difficult to consider themselves worthy of reviewing products authored by more senior physicians and scientists. Peer reviewers early in their career may also discover it difficult to provide critical feedback or reject a manuscript given their personal experience in receiving such responses from editors themselves. And if critical feedback is required, reviewers may find it a challenge to frame these often difficult comments in a collegial and educational manner. Fortunate are the earlier career faculty who have a mentor who is willing to guide the novice reviewer through his or her first peer review assignments.

Publication Process

The submission of a manuscript to a journal is the start of a long process in which the work is judged on its clinical and scientific merits and suitability for publication. The peer reviewer is but one part of this editorial progression. When a manuscript is first submitted, which is now most commonly done through an online process, it is reviewed by the editor or an associate editor to ensure that the author(s) followed the journal's instructions and whether the paper is appropriate in scope and science for the journal's readership. If these criteria are satisfied, the editorial office then focuses on identifying the appropriate individuals for peer review of the submitted product.

A reviewer may be identified for any number of reasons. Reviewers are often considered experts in the subject matter of the manuscript. In addition, reviewers with a history of providing timely, quality reviews are often chosen by editorial offices for their proven insight. To help identify worthy reviewers, most journals maintain a database of identified experts in various fields of study, as well individuals who have previously reviewed for the journal. It is from this list that the editorial office attempts to select the most qualified peer reviewer for the manuscript in question. It is in the journal editors' best interest to identify careful, thorough, timely, and fair reviewers to help judge and improve submitted manuscripts. Editors may also identify reviewers with differing scientific and clinical strengths to review a single submission. For example, one reviewer may be selected who specializes in the clinical care of the population discussed in a manuscript while another reviewer may be knowledgeable in the unique scientific method or statistics used in the study. Editors rarely invite reviewers who are not appropriate or up to the requested task. Journals vary in the time allotted to reviewers and also have differing standards on the number of peer reviewers required to review each manuscript. Journal editors have attempted over the years to develop a manuscript review process that is fair for the author and peer reviewer.

After reviewers are selected by the editors, they receive an e-mail inviting them to review the manuscript. The e-mail often contains the editor's invitation to review, the manuscript's title and abstract, along with the author list (unless a blind process is used), and an approximate review due date. In the e-mail, the potential reviewer will be given the options to accept or decline the invitation to review. If the invitation is accepted, the reviewer will be directed to the journal's manuscript site for an electronic copy of the manuscript to be reviewed along with the required review forms. Once the editorial office has received all the reviews, the editor assesses the feedback and recommendations provided by the reviewers. He or she will then make a decision on the disposition of the manuscript and draft a letter to the authors, outlining this decision along with the reviewers' comments to the authors.

Questions to Ask Oneself When Asked to Review a Manuscript

There are several questions that prospective peer reviewers may want to pose to themselves before embarking on the requested review (see Table 12.1) [3]. First, does the reviewer have some conflict of interest with the manuscript in question that may interfere with the ability to provide an unbiased opinion to the journal's editors? It is the reviewer's obligation to avoid any potential conflicts of interest that may contaminate the peer review process. If a potential reviewer has any questions about a potential conflict of interest, it is best to query the editorial office with the particulars of the perceived conflict. If the solicited peer reviewer feels that there is a conflict of interest and cannot provide a balanced and fair view of the manuscript, the reviewer should respectfully decline the review offer.

The second question prospective reviewers should ask themselves is whether the manuscript's content (topic or science) falls outside the reviewer's area of expertise. A poor understanding of the article's topic may fundamentally hamper the ability of the reviewer to adequately evaluate the manuscript. Lovejoy et al. [4] recommend that reviewers, early in their academic career, choose no more than three areas of expertise in which they will review manuscripts. These areas should include topics in which they have authored peer-reviewed manuscripts and/or conducted research. By narrowing the scope of expertise early, one is able to focus on providing quality reviews and building a reputation as a skilled reviewer. Additional areas of expertise may be established in future years.

Table 12.1 Questions the potePublication:process, manuscript submission: potential reviewer questionsntial reviewer should ask when invited to review [9]

1. Do I have enough expertise in the content of this manuscript to provide a fair and competent review?
2. Do I have sufficient time to perform a meaningful review of the manuscript within the requested time frame?
3. Do I have any potential conflicts of interest that may bias my perception of this manuscript?

Last, but not least in the minds of early career academic faculty, is whether or not they have the time to complete the requested review. The prospective reviewer needs to be certain that he or she can perform a quality review, in addition to all other academic and clinical obligations, before agreeing to the editor's offer to review a manuscript. If invited reviewers are uncertain to whether they can produce a useful review within the allotted time frame, it is best to decline the review request.

Whatever the reason for the denial, the editorial office should be notified soon after the invitation to review is received. This prompt denial will allow the editorial office to identify another prospective peer to review the manuscript. Editors usually await the reviews from all peer referees before notifying the authors of the manuscript's status; it is therefore important to be respectful of the provided deadline for returning the peer review. This timeliness is imperative to maintain a smooth publication process and to avoid antagonizing anxious authors awaiting word on the fate of their submitted manuscripts.

What Makes a Good Reviewer?

It is important to note that there are no clear predictors of which peer reviewers produce the best quality manuscript reviews [5]. In a study by Black et al. [6], the characteristics of reviewers had little relationship with the quality of the reviews produced. The only significant factor associated with reviews rated higher in quality was when the reviewer had received training in statistics or epidemiology. Goldbeck-Wood et al. [7] felt that professional idealism, intellectual curiosity, and punctuality were important qualities for successful peer reviewers. Taking part in the peer review process allows one a special, albeit confidential, insight into new knowledge and technological breakthroughs. In addition, by reviewing the manuscripts of others, one may improve one's own academic work. Reviewers must have intellectual curiosity and a desire to educate others towards the betterment of science to produce meaningful reviews.

How to Review a Scientific Manuscript

Preparation

Once the invitation to review has been accepted, the process of serving as a peer reviewer truly begins. Time management is an important part of the review process. The time required depends on the reviewer and the manuscript under review and, therefore, varies considerably. One survey revealed that the mean time reviewers spent on a review was 3 h [8]. Although the reviewer often has expertise in the subject manner of the manuscript, it may be helpful to perform a literature search on the topic under discussion to update and help frame the paper's subject manner.

Quick Read

The brief literature review is followed by a quick read through of the manuscript to appreciate the overall quality and character of the work. In extreme cases this initial read may provide enough insight into the significant flaws of the manuscript to lead the reviewer to recommend rejection. However, in a vast majority of cases, this early read allows reviewers to familiarize themselves with the goals and scope of the paper. Have the authors succeeded in clearly stating and justifying their purpose for writing the manuscript? The reviewer also starts to form an opinion about the manuscript's appropriateness for the journal for which it is being considered for publication. It may be helpful to read the journal's mission statement when determining the suitability of a submitted manuscript for a specific journal [9]. If not clearly stated in the invitation to review the manuscript, the initial read of the manuscript allows the reviewer to think about in which category the article belongs; is it a clinical study, basic science study, a clinical review, or a case report? It is important to know whether the journal publishes the type of manuscript you have identified. This information can usually be found in the journal's instructions to potential authors.

Hard/Critical Read

If the reviewer thinks the manuscript has some merit, it is time for the more thorough and critical manuscript read. The purpose of these subsequent reads is to comment on all aspects of the paper and provide the editor and author with specific feedback on how to improve the manuscript. The goal of this feedback is to improve the quality of the manuscript and ideally to make it worthy of publication eventually.

At this point of the process, the reviewer focuses on the significance of the question posed by the authors, along with the originality and rationale of the approach used to answer that question. It is also at this time that the data are carefully reviewed, along with the quality and significance of results garnered from that data. These subsequent critical reads allow the reviewer to fulfill his or her responsibility to carefully evaluate all components of the manuscript, provide specific feedback on these elements, and convey his or her objective, general impression of the worthiness of the manuscript for publication. The specifics of this review will be discussed in the following sections.

Introduction

In the introduction of an article the authors need to convey the importance of the topic of the manuscript. There needs to be a clear statement of the clinical problem or research question that the manuscript is going to address [10]. The authors need to show that the article is both relevant and important to the journal's readership. This is often best accomplished through a brief literature review, which summarizes the current state of the science. The literature chosen should be focused, but objective and fair, as it attempts to help justify the conduct of the study or stress the importance of the clinical topic undergoing review.

Methods/Statistics

The methods section should be evaluated for the completeness and clarity of the methodological processes utilized in the study or literature review. The methods section needs to show the reviewers that the study is valid. In research manuscripts this is accomplished by a clear description of the study design, procedures, ethical safeguards, and means of data analyses. The research design should be sufficiently described and detailed to allow the study to be replicated [11]. The authors' methods and data analysis must be sound and appropriate for the research question. If there are flaws in the methods, the validity and generalizability of a study suffer.

Unless there are flagrant errors, reviewers should assume that the data provided are valid [12]. Journal editors do not expect that all reviewers are experts in statistical analysis. They do, however, expect that reviewers are familiar with some basic knowledge of statistics [8]. The rationale for the statistical analysis in the manuscript, along with the analysis itself, needs to be comprehensible to the journal's readership. If the reviewer is unclear on the statistical techniques employed in the study or questions the analysis itself, it is appropriate to request that the editor identifies a statistical consultant or another peer reviewer more familiar with the statistical analysis. If this help is required, it is useful to notify the editorial office early in the review to avoid unnecessarily delaying the process.

Results

The results section of the paper should be complete and well organized. Some information conveyed in the text may be better displayed in the form of a table or figure. If data are presented in a figure or table, they should not be repeated in their entirety within the text. The results need to be presented in a manner so that their relationship to the research problem is clearly understood by the reader. It is also important that the results are consistent in all sections of the paper.

Conclusion/Discussion

The review of the discussion section should focus on the authors' ability to adequately interpret the findings of the study. In doing so the authors should carefully frame the main findings of the work in the context of the research question. The paper's results should be compared and contrasted to the current state of the science through a literature search. The reviewer will also need to determine if the author's conclusions are adequately supported by the manuscript's findings.

Reviewers should determine if the authors have adequately identified and discussed the strengths and limitations of the research. If alternative explanations of the paper's findings are possible, these alternatives should be objectively explored and discussed by the authors. The theoretical implications of the study's results should be discussed in this section, along with a comment on any potential future research questions that may be informed by the results of the present study [11].

Abstract/Title

A well-written abstract and title are imperative to a successful and well-referenced article. If the title is not appropriately catchy and the abstract does not adequately present the paper's content, it is quite possible that few will read the manuscript. This fact is all the more true in the age of electronic literature searches in which the title and abstract are quickly accessed for review, but to access the full article often requires additional steps. By saving the review of the paper's abstract and title, until now the reviewer can better appreciate the contents and significance of the manuscript. This understanding of the manuscript helps ensure that the relevant information is summarized, represented, and highlighted in the title and abstract.

Some journals have a specific abstract format that authors are required to use to ensure that all the relevant parts of the abstract are included in the submission. In addition, there should be no inconsistencies between the information included in the abstract and the data discussed in the text. Despite the apparent simplicity of this statement, inconsistencies have been found. Pitkin et al. [13] reviewed 44 abstracts from each of six different journals and found that 18–68 % of the abstracts from the various journals contained data that were inconsistent or absent from the main body of the manuscript.

Illustrations

There are many different types of illustrations in the medical literature. The most common include tables, graphs, and algorithms, but authors may also include imaging studies, drawings, and pictures. Illustrations, whatever the format, should always enhance the message of the text, not simply repeat information already provided elsewhere in the manuscript. Tables and graphs often accomplish this by allowing for improved organization and comparison of data. Algorithms may be helpful in elucidating the research protocol, describing a proposed treatment protocol, or outlining an administrative structure. If information is presented in tables, figures, or algorithms, it should not be repeated in the text. Rather, the text should be used to describe and highlight the key elements in the data detailed in the figure [14].

Illustrations are often best used to convey information that is optimally communicated visually rather than in text format. This often allows for improved understanding as well as limiting word count. For example, artist representations or pictures are often used as an effective means of communicating medical or surgical techniques. Information provided in the illustration, whatever the format, must agree with the data in the manuscript's text. The illustrations should also be of sufficient technical quality to allow for reader interpretation. And finally, the legends must match the illustrations and be adequately descriptive of the illustration's content.

References

The references are usually the last part of a manuscript reviewed. The reviewer, given his or her relative expertise in the subject of the manuscript, should have an appreciation of the state of the literature. This should help the reviewer appreciate if the references are current, balanced, and relevant. The reviewer should also make sure no important and pertinent references have been omitted by the authors. If a reference is cited, it should be accurately represented in the text. The references in the manuscript should be used to give credit appropriately to ideas and findings discussed in the text. A majority of references should be from peer-reviewed primary sources as opposed to secondary sources (e.g., textbooks) [15].

Readability

It is not the reviewer's responsibility to correct grammar or spelling. The journal's staff will address most of the common grammatical errors found in submission once the manuscript is accepted for publication. The peer reviewer, however, needs to ensure that the manuscript flows logically and reads easily. If the writing is so poor as to interfere with the reader's basic understanding and appreciation of the article, it is appropriate to return the manuscript to the editor and confidentially suggest that it be rewritten before further consideration for publication [8].

Conflict of Interests/IRB/Plagiarism Concerns

All manuscript authors are required to disclose potential conflicts of interest. The reviewer should notify the editorial office if he or she identifies any non-declared conflicts of interest that could adversely affect the credibility of the manuscript under review. If appropriate to the type of study, an explicit statement of approval by a suitable institutional review board (IRB) should be included in the manuscript. Lastly, if the reviewer identifies a concern for plagiarism or any other lapse in scholarly integrity, he or she should notify the editor promptly in a confidential manner.

Reviewer Responsibilities

The peer reviewer has multiple important obligations to ensure that the publication process moves smoothly and that high standards of scientific conduct are maintained. These responsibilities include maintaining confidentiality, managing potential conflicts of interest, and preserving a collegial academic approach to the review process. The manuscript under review needs to be treated as a confidential, privileged communication. The existence and contents of the manuscript should not be disclosed as it is the intellectual property of the authors [16]. The reviewer should never contact the author of a manuscript under review; all communication should take place through the journal's editorial office. As mentioned earlier, if the reviewer believes that there is the potential for a conflict of interest related to his or her involvement in the review process, he or she should refuse the opportunity to review the manuscript. Possible conflicts of interest may include personal, professional, or financial interests with a variety of individuals, corporations, or institutions related to the publication. If there is no reviewer conflict of interest, this should be documented in the comments to the editor.

One of the foremost responsibilities of the peer reviewer is to educate in a professional and collegial manner. The goal of the review process is to improve the science, the manuscript, and the profession. These noble goals are best accomplished by the reviewer when he or she provides comments in as constructive and empathetic manner as possible. A vast majority of reviewers have authored papers and can therefore relate to how easy it is to become defensive when critical feedback is provided on one's work. A careful, consistent, and considerate approach to criticism by the reviewer is therefore appropriate. It is imperative that the peer reviewer, after agreeing to review the manuscript, completes the assigned task in the allotted time. If reviewers do not feel that they will be able to meet the deadline, they should update the editorial office to this fact. These responsibilities of the peer reviewer are important and affect the author, editor, and the journal.

Review Forms

Most journals employ a web-based manuscript submission and review system. Although there is no universal peer review form, most are fairly similar in the structure and the information requested from the peer reviewer. The editors want to know if the manuscript is appropriate for the journal, if any conflicts of interests have been identified, or if the scientific question is worthy of publication. These common structured questions are usually answered in the web-based systems with a simple point-and-click, yes–no response. Most peer review systems also request that the reviewer provides specific feedback to the editor (in confidence) and to the manuscript's authors. The written feedback provided to the editor and to the authors should be constructive and consistent in narrative.

Comments to the Editor

The reviewer's comments to the editor are entered into a specific section of the review form. These comments are a confidential communication between the reviewer and editor. They are not shared with the author. This is the place to comment on the strengths and weaknesses of the paper, request statistical consultation, and/or raise issues with the paper that may not be appropriate to communicate with the authors (e.g., concern of plagiarism). Most journals will also request that the reviewer makes a recommendation about whether the paper should be published as submitted. The reviewer's educated recommendation is part of the decision process, but the editor will make the final determination on the status of the manuscript. Reviewers, therefore, should not be offended if the editor's decision differs from their recommendation.

The reviewer's comments to the editor usually begin with a brief synopsis of the manuscript. This summary usually runs a couple of sentences and identifies the topic, research approach, significant findings, and conclusions [4]. This is followed by detailed descriptions of the article's strengths and weaknesses. The editor should be made aware of the importance and timelessness of the manuscript, the relevance of the article to the journal's readership, and the appropriateness of the study design. The reviewer should also provide the editor with comments on how the authors may improve the manuscript. If deficits are identified in the study design and methods, improper data analysis techniques were used, or faulty conclusions were drawn from the results, these need to be mentioned. In addition, if the reviewer finds poor grammar, inappropriately vague language, bias, and/or improper interpretation of a literature citation, these also need to be communicated to the editor. The reviewer, however, should not get bogged down in minor grammatical errors but, rather, focus on mistakes that decrease the general readability of the manuscript. For each of the weaknesses identified, it is helpful for the reviewer to acknowledge what the authors may be able to do to correct the deficiency. If the reviewer has previously received permission from the editor to share the reviewer duties with others, that is acknowledged in this section as well [17].

The reviewer then has the opportunity to make a recommendation regarding the disposition of the manuscript. The reviewer is often given a choice of recommendations regarding the publication readiness of the manuscript: reject, accept pending revision (major or minor), or accept (see Table 12.2). When the reviewer provides this recommendation, he or she is weighing the paper's strengths and weaknesses and differentiating minor concerns from fatal flaws. Whatever the suggestion, it needs to be consistent with the comments provided to the editor and author. All decisions about final acceptance or rejection of the manuscript rest with the editor. These editorial decisions are based upon criteria of significance and quality. The editor determines these criteria based on his or her personal opinion of the manuscript as well as the comments and recommendations received from all the reviewers.

Table 12.2 Recommendations for manuscript disposition

Accept the manuscript

The recommendation to accept a manuscript implies that the paper is ready for publication but may require some minor editorial work

- It is appropriate for the journal's readership
- It adds something of value to the current literature
- It contains no scientific flaws
- The conclusion is appropriate
- It is without ethical concerns
- It is well written
- Its references are appropriate

Revise the manuscript

The recommendation that an author revises a manuscript implies that it has value and is important to publish but requires some work by the author to improve identified areas of deficiency

- It is appropriate for the journal's readership
- It adds something of value to the current literature
- It contains no significant scientific flaws which cannot be addressed upon reanalysis or revision
- The conclusion, while valid, may require some mild reinterpretation or clarification
- It is without ethical concerns
- It may require some editing to improve flow and/or clarity
- Its references may require strengthening

(continued)

Table 12.2 (continued)

Reject the manuscript

The recommendation to reject a manuscript communicates to the author(s) that the manuscript is inappropriate for the journal in which it has been submitted for publication. Depending on the flaw, any one of the following may be sufficient for the recommendation of outright rejection of a manuscript

- It is not appropriate for the journal's readership
- It does not add something of value to the current literature
- It contains significant scientific flaws
- The conclusion is not valid
- It contains ethical concerns
- It is poorly written
- Its references are not appropriate

Comments to the Author

In contrast to the comments to the editor, the comments provided to the author are meant to be shared with the editor and the manuscript's author(s). Most journals mask the reviewer's identity to the authors receiving the feedback. These anonymous comments to authors are the most valuable part of the review. It is here that the reviewer provides the authors with the honest feedback necessary to improve the manuscript with the idea of advancing the science and educational merit of the publication. It is also in this section that the information to substantiate the confidential recommendation to the editor to reject, revise, or accept should be provided to the author. The facts in this section must correlate well with the information provided to the editors to avoid unnecessary confusion between editor and author. The reviewer needs to maintain a collegial and professional tone in this section. The goal is to educate and improve the manuscript, not to disparage and denigrate the authors.

Similar to the comments in the editor section, the comments in the author section should ideally be composed of an introductory paragraph and specific comments about the paper's value, strengths, and weaknesses, followed by a concluding paragraph. The reviewer's opinion on acceptance or rejection of the manuscript should not be included in the comments to the authors. It is often helpful for the reviewer to organize his or her constructive comments on the strengths and weaknesses of the paper by following the paper's structure (e.g., introduction, methods, results, conclusion). It may also be useful to number each suggestion, which may allow a more effective author response and review of the manuscript's revision.

The brief introduction paragraph, which summarizes the paper's objective, methodology, findings, and conclusions, demonstrates to the authors that you have read the paper and understand its content and premise. This is often copied directly from the comments to the editor. This paragraph is ideally followed by a section-by-section, detailed description of the paper's strengths and weaknesses, for example, comments on the clarity and brevity of the abstract or the generalizability of the results. Be specific and give examples. The more precise the comments, the more likely the authors are to incorporate them into the revision of the manuscript. Each weakness should be clearly elucidated and never left as a general, unsupported, and qualitative statement. In addition, suggestions on various ways the authors may address the identified weakness should be included when possible. The goal is for the authors to use the information provided in these reviewer comments to better understand the editor's publication decision and eventually improve the manuscript.

Types of Manuscripts

Many types of manuscripts are submitted for publication, and each is meant to provide the reader with a different type of necessary information. They are each written with a different purpose in mind and therefore require a slightly different method of peer review. The reviewer should be aware if the journal they are reviewing for accepts only specific types of manuscripts. Journals may also provide detailed formatting instructions for various types of manuscripts. It is therefore important for the reviewer to be familiar with these instructions to authors, which are most often located on the journal's website.

Case Reports

Case reports may be suitable for publication if they provide important new information that offers a unique understanding of a specific illness [8]. The report should include information detailed enough to allow the reader to diagnose or treat the patient in question. Case reports should be considered for publication if there is something truly unique about the case and/or treatment. The report should also add to the literature, educate the reader, and have the potential to improve patient care. The structure, clarity, and flow of a case report are very important and should be commented on by the reviewer.

> **Key Concepts**
> - Be polite and respectful.
> - Be prompt in responses and deliver reviews on time.
> - Be consistent in comments and recommendations.
> - Be ethical and unbiased.
> - Be knowledgeable in what you review.

Clinical Research

Regardless of the type of research study performed, the evaluation of the manuscript starts with the validity of the research question. Once the validity of the question is assessed, the reviewer must turn his or her attention to the means in which the authors sought to answer this question. The researchers need to be clear about what type of study is being reported and provide a description of their research population and sampling procedures. If applicable, the methods section should also include a clear confirmation that the study was approved by an IRB and the steps taken to protect the study population clearly delineated. The data gathered needs to be assessed, which may require the use of a statistical consultant assigned through the editorial office of the journal. The conclusion of the paper needs to align with the results. There should also be a careful and focused discussion about how the results of the present study fit within current scientific knowledge or clinical practice.

Reviews

In assessing a clinical review article, it is important to understand how its publication would benefit the journal's readership. A review article might, for example, summarize the development of a new treatment for an old clinical problem. A review article could also import relevant knowledge available in other literature to the journal readers who are not usually exposed to that information (e.g., geriatric medicine's literature on delirium prevention reviewed for an orthopedic surgery journal). Whereas the author's expertise and knowledge about the manuscript's topic should be clear when reviewing a review article, there should be no evidence of authorship bias. A review article must present a balanced, inclusive, and objective look at the current state of the literature. This requires the reviewer to check the references for potential important omissions and the use of primary sources.

Reviewing a Revision

If the journal's editors request that the authors revise and resubmit the manuscript, the revision will usually be forwarded to the original reviewer for reassessment. The authors should include a cover letter outlining all the changes made to the manuscript. Ideally these changes will be referenced to the suggestions provided by the peer reviewers and editors during the initial review process. The reviewer needs to determine if the authors have adequately addressed the concerns raised on the previous review. It is not appropriate at this stage for the reviewer to raise new concerns. At the conclusion of this rereview, the reviewer will again be asked for his or her opinion on a disposition of the manuscript.

Conclusion

The peer review process is the current standard for assessing a manuscript's worthiness for publication in the scientific literature. Reviewers, therefore, serve a critical role in ensuring the dissemination of knowledge throughout the medical profession. The entire peer review process is based on the idealism, professionalism, and collegiality of the peer reviewer (see Table 12.3). Peer reviewers provide fair, constructive, and knowledgeable feedback on a manuscript that improves the quality of the manuscript and aids the editor in determining an appropriate disposition of the manuscript. Accepting an invitation to review demonstrates a willingness to contribute to the profession of medicine and the advancement of knowledge.

Table 12.3 Professionalism in peer review [3]

Reviewers must
1. Manage manuscripts that they are reviewing as a privileged and confidential document
2. Review only manuscripts that fall within their scope of expertise
3. Maintain a collegial and helpful tone when providing feedback
4. Uphold high ethical standards (i.e., disclose potential conflicts of interest, avoid bias)

Words to the Wise
- Request feedback from editors on the quality of your submitted reviews.
- Ask the editorial office if they would be willing to share the comments from the other reviewers involved in the review of the manuscript.
- With the permission of the editor, seek permission to review a manuscript with a more senior faculty mentor.
- Treat the authors of the manuscript you are reviewing as you, as a fellow author, would like to be treated by the reviewers of your manuscripts.

Ask Your Mentor or Colleagues
- How does an early-career faculty member get invited to review manuscripts?
- When I get the opportunity to review along with permission from the journal's editorial office, could you please provide feedback on the quality of my review?
- How does a peer reviewer provide critical comments to the manuscript's author(s) in a constructive and respectful manner?
- How many reviews should I do a year?

References

1. Kronick DA. Peer review in 18th-century scientific journalism. JAMA. 1990;263(10):1321–2.
2. Bordage G, Caelleigh AS. A tool for reviewers: Review criteria for research manuscripts. Acad Med. 2001;76(9):904–8.
3. Roberts LW, Coverdale J, Edenharder K, et al. How to review a manuscript; a "down-to-earth" approach. Acad Psychiatry. 2004;28(2):81–5.
4. Lovejoy TI, Revenson TA, France CR. Reviewing manuscripts for peer-review journals: A primer for novice and seasoned reviewers. Ann Behav Med. 2011;42:1–13.
5. Alexandrov AV, Hennerici MG, Norrving B. Suggestions for reviewing manuscripts. Cerebrovasc Dis. 2009;28:243–6.
6. Black N, van Rooyen S, Godlee F, et al. What makes a good reviewer and a good review for a general medical journal? JAMA. 1998;280:231–3.
7. Goldbeck-Wood S. Evidence on peer review-scientific quality control or smokescreen? BMJ. 1999;318:44–5.
8. McNutt RA, Evans AT, Fletcher RH, et al. The effects of blinding on the quality of peer review. A randomized trial. JAMA. 1990;263(10):1371–6.
9. Rosenfeld RM. How to review journal manuscripts. Otolaryngol Head Neck Surg. 2010;142(4):472–86.
10. McGaghie WC, Bordage G, Shea JA. Problem statement, conceptual framework, and research question. Acad Med. 2001;76(9):923–4.
11. McGaghie WC, Bordage G, Crandall S, et al. Research design. Acad Med. 2001;76(9):929–30.
12. Levine AM, Heckman JD, Hensinger RN. The art and science of reviewing manuscripts for orthopaedic journals: part II. Optimizing the manuscript: practical hints for improving the quality of reviews. Instr Course Lect. 2004;53:689–97.

13. Pitkin RM, Branagan MA, Burmeister LF. Accuracy of data in abstracts of published research articles. JAMA. 1999;281(12):1110–1.
14. Regehr G. Presentation of results. Acad Med. 2001;76(9):940–2.
15. Christenbery TL. Manuscript peer review: a guide for advanced practice nurses. J Am Acad Nurse Pract. 2011;23(1):15–22.
16. Salasche SJ. How to "peer review" a medical journal manuscript. Dermatol Surg. 1997;23(6):423–8.
17. Hoppin FG. How I review an original scientific article. Am J Respir Crit Care Med. 2002;166:1019–23.

How to Understand Flaws in Clinical Research

13

Teddy D. Warner

Health researchers, providers, consumers, and policy makers are confronted with unmanageable amounts of information. Being able to understand flaws that commonly arise in clinical research is an essential skill for academic faculty in clinical departments. There are a number of important issues or problems that seriously limit one's ability to trust the published outcomes in clinical research (Table 13.1) as authoritative.

First, quantitative researchers often examine tightly *defined questions* without first considering a broader view in defining a problem. In contrast, qualitative researchers usually take a much broader view initially than do quantitative researchers, but qualitative researchers do not conduct controlled trials of efficacy or effectiveness. Qualitative researchers seek to thoroughly explore the nature and extent of a problem or issue without being constrained by the need to reduce their results to numbers and statistics or having to predefine the specific scope of what they are studying. Qualitative researchers seek to have their data and interpretations of their findings show them the way to understanding. In contrast, clinical researchers may rely on broad epidemiological

T.D. Warner, Ph.D. (✉)
Department of Family and Community Medicine, University of New Mexico School of Medicine, Albuquerque, NM, USA
e-mail: twarner@salud.unm.edu

© Springer International Publishing Switzerland 2016   191
L.W. Roberts (ed.), *The Clinician Educator Guidebook*,
DOI 10.1007/978-3-319-27980-0_13

Table 13.1 Some general criteria for evaluating clinical research study outcome validity

1. What are the main *objectives* of the study and are they clearly and completely specified? Will meeting the objectives advance meaningful knowledge in the field or subfield?
2. What is the *type of study* (e.g., randomized trial, nonrandomized trial, nonequivalent control group, case control, case cohort, cross-sectional descriptive, qualitative)? Is the design clearly and completely described? What is the basic *research design* and is it clearly and completed specified? (a) Descriptive (e.g., case studies, observations, simple survey, interviews, focus groups) (b) Relational or correlational or associative (e.g., complex self-report or survey) (c) Comparative or case control (i.e., preexisting equivalent or nonequivalent groups) (d) Quasi-experimental (i.e., nonrandomized assignment) (e) Experimental (i.e., randomized assignment) (f) Review (i.e., narrative, systematic, meta-analytic)
3. Does the *Introduction* adequately place the study in the proper context the literature that is centrally important to the study? Recognize that only studies directly pertinent to the study objectives are expected to be discussed. Determine what important and uncited studies, if any, do *not* inform this study and how that may have influenced the study design, conduct, and reporting
4. What are the *primary hypotheses*, if any, and are they clearly stated in a *testable form*? Are there secondary hypotheses? Are the hypotheses reasonably justified and significant to the field? Note that exploratory or purely descriptive studies may well not have hypotheses, but most other studies should have them
5. Were the hypotheses based on a theory or conceptual model? If not, is an atheoretical approach overtly justified by the authors?
6. Is the design adequate to meet study objectives and answer study hypotheses? Objectives, hypotheses, and design should be consonant with each other
7. What *population* was sampled for the study? What is the theoretical population of interest (i.e., to whom do the researchers ideally wish to generalize their conclusions)? How was the *sample* drawn (e.g., randomly, purposively, self-selected)? Does the sample allow generalization to a population of real interest?

(continued)

Table 13.1 (continued)

8. If the approach is comparative, quasi-experimental, or experimental, what is the *full study design* in terms of independent or predictor variables? For example, is there more than a single independent or predictor variable (IV)?

9. What are the main *independent* or *predictor* variables (if it is not purely a descriptive study)? Are the independent variables important or peripheral to the phenomenon under study? Are independent or predictor variables manipulated by the researchers or are they only measured as attributes of participants? Is the independent variable a *between subjects* variable (represented by different groups of individuals) or a *within subjects* variable [variables repeatedly measured at different points in time, most commonly, or measures from different sources that are correlated (e.g., from husbands and wives as pairs, or repeated measures from subjects)]?

10. Are these variables justified from the extant literature, and are all key such variables included in some way in the design (i.e., is the study analytic model fully specified based on what is known)?

11. What is the *level of measurement* of the predictor and *independent* variables (*nominal/categorical*, *ordinal*, *interval/continuous*, or *ratio/continuous*), and are the analyses appropriate for that level of measurement?

12. What is the main *dependent* or *outcome* variable(s)? What is the level of measurement of the dependent or outcome variable(s) (*nominal/categorical*, *ordinal*, *interval/continuous*, or *ratio/continuous*), and is the analysis suitable for that level of measurement?

13. Are the primary outcomes conceptually appropriate, given the extant literature about the phenomenon studied? Are there also secondary outcomes which are less central to the effects of the independent or predictor variable? Were the most conceptually important outcomes assessed, or were key outcomes omitted?

14. Is there sufficient evidence for the *reliability* of the main outcome variables [no evidence vs. provided by past literature based on citations vs. provided by the data in the present study (always preferable)]? (Note that reliability of measures is sample-dependent and is a *feature of the data* acquired and *not* of the instrument used to measure the outcomes)

15. What level of control (i.e., *randomization*, *stratification*, *equivalent groups*, *statistical control*) is exerted in the study over *extraneous variables* (i.e., variables other than the independent/predictor and dependent/outcome variables)? Do any important uncontrolled extraneous variables produce possible *confounds* with the independent or predictor variables that might provide plausible alternative explanations for study results?

(continued)

Table 13.1 (continued)

---

16. If *statistical control* (i.e., in regression or ANCOVA models) is used for extraneous variables (i.e., covariates), were the interaction effects of the covariate with the study independent variables and other covariates formally tested for presence? Analysis of covariance assumes the covariate does not interact with other model predictors, but if it does, then failure to include the covariate X predictor interaction term in the model may fully invalidate results obtained for study outcomes

---

17. Does the *Methods* section adequately describe key features of the study such that the study could be replicated by others and that readers can fairly assess the likely validity of reported outcomes?

---

18. At the outset of the study, are *groups* (if any) that are compared in the study equivalent or different on important characteristics (i.e., can preexisting characteristics or conditions explain or confound the study results)?

---

19. What is the *dropout or incompletion rate* of study participants, and does this vary by study group? How does this compare to other studies of its type using similar approaches? What *analytic model* was applied to deal with incomplete data (e.g., intent to treat, as normally preferred or some other method)?

---

20. How were *missing data* dealt with (e.g., ignored, cases dropped, simple imputation methods, state-of-the-art imputation methods), and how could that process influence study outcomes and validity of effects detected?

---

21. Did sufficient numbers of study participants complete the final study outcomes to provide adequate statistical power? Is *sufficient statistical power* present to detect the *smallest effect sizes* that are *clinically meaningful*? How were sample sizes determined? Is there *excessive study power* (i.e., a very large sample) that is likely to produce statistically significant differences for clinically trivial or unimportant effect sizes? What is the *minimum clinically significant difference* (MCID) for the phenomenon studied, and is that reported and discussed for this study?

---

22. Are appropriate *statistical procedures* applied to the data? Were important assumptions for these procedures tested and met (e.g., uniformity of regression for all groups on all covariates, absence of interactions effects that are not included in the final model, independence of observations)? Would alternative or additional statistical procedures enhance the ability to understand results?

---

23. Does the *Results* section clearly and succinctly describe all important results in the study based on the objectives and hypotheses? Were clear and informative *tables* and *figures* for data included? Would additional figures or tables enhance interpretation of study results?

(continued)

Table 13.1   (continued)

24. Does the *Discussion* section clearly and succinctly summarize:
    (a) The major results from the study, while placing them in perspective to current knowledge
    (b) The important implications of the study results
    (c) The important limitations of the study
    (d) Specific needed directions for future research

25. Are the study results *appropriately interpreted* (i.e., was interpretation justified by the nature of the measures, how they were obtained, who they were obtained from, and how they were analyzed)? Were conclusions appropriate or overstated or incomplete or misleading?

26. Do the study results contribute to the existing *knowledge base* (i.e., current relevant empirical literature) incrementally? If not, is the study so novel that it provides unique information, and if so, is this clearly stated? Do the study results replicate or contradict important previous findings? What practical or theoretical relevance do study results and outcomes have?

27. Are all *citations* included in the body of the article cited in the Reference list? Are they cited in standard fashion such that they could easily be located in the literature?

28. Based on an *overall evaluation* of the article, does the research seem valid? Do you believe the outcomes, conclusions, and implications? If not, what is your *rationale* for disbelieving?

29. What is the *next research* that should follow from this work, and was that described and explained by the authors?

data about a phenomenon of interest or its importance, but they often then define a narrow range of subject characteristics, a limited population, and only a single outcome to measure.

All of these factors combine to limit the possibility of the study to show valid results. Null results under such conditions may well fail to generate information about relationships or causes simply because of the narrow scope of all the factors in the study. That is, a broader range for the variables studied may have revealed statistically significant and clinically meaningful effects or relationships. This type of problem is sometimes called a "restriction of range" problem. Without studying the broader set of factors and degrees of each factor, a researcher may never know why his or her study failed to detect effects and the value of the study may not be as great in advancing a field of scientific inquiry.

Second, researchers often conduct studies in *artificial and highly controlled settings*. In experimental studies, researchers do their best to control all variables other than the independent variables directly being studied to determine if they cause variation in the outcomes or dependent variables. In such highly controlled circumstances, other naturally occurring variables in the real world may be prevented from having their normal effects on outcomes. Controlled settings and studies are needed, however, because conducting research in uncontrolled real-world settings might well lead to results that would be difficult to interpret because of the operation of many influential, confounding variables that might interact with the study's independent variables. In short, researchers often must trade off efforts in studying variables in complex, real-world situations vs. studying them in controlled and artificial settings, which may produce more interpretable results about cause and effects, at least in the early stages of studying a phenomenon. In many research situations, after highly controlled laboratory studies have shown that the independent variables cause variation in outcome variables (efficacy), a researcher may then shift to conducting a related study in more natural environments to determine if the laboratory results generalize to real-world settings and under what circumstances they apply (effectiveness). That is, controlled RCTs usually need to be followed by translational studies to actual practice settings. In most cases, translational studies have not yet been performed and reported, and because of this NIH has greatly increased its emphasis on various phases of translational research [1].

Third, researchers often use highly *imperfect measures that show low reliability*, often unknowingly. Just as all studies are imperfect to varying degrees, all *measures* of outcomes are also imperfect. Many factors can contribute to error in measurements. Measures with a lot of error have lower reliability than measures with less error, and measures with lower reliability have lower validity as a result of lower measurement consistency. Thus, researchers generally should strive to make measurements as accurate and reliable as feasible. More reliable and more valid measures have greater statistical power to detect relationships with other variables, thus they increase the likelihood that a study will support its hypotheses if the predicted relationships or effects actually occur in the population being studied [2]. So, proper assessment of a study must consider the quality of the measures used in the work.

Fourth, researchers often *use far less than ideal samples* that prevent generalization to the true population of interest. Generalizability of outcomes is also termed the *external validity* of the outcomes. To have confidence in the generalizability of study outcomes, the sample should at least be *representative* of the population of interest. Realize that if a study's outcomes do not generalize to any broader population of importance than the study sample, then the study results are not very useful or meaningful. Of course, in most cases, generalizability can only be fully confirmed by replication of study outcomes in future studies, engaging diverse samples acquired from diverse populations. This said, a study sample demonstrated to be representative on key variables with the population may suggest that study outcomes are likely to be generalizable.

Ideally, a sample should be randomly drawn from the population. In health-related research, few samples are randomly drawn due to practical constraints. Most samples do not even end up being representative of the larger population of interest (e.g., all individuals with some type of disorder), and characteristics of individuals in study samples are very often quite unrepresentative of the population. Instead, most researchers draw samples of convenience (i.e., samples relevant and accessible to the researcher), which helps accomplish the work but affects the generalization of study outcomes. The unrepresentativeness of a sample may well be the reason that the study outcomes do not replicate in future work that involves different samples of individuals.

Fifth, researchers usually conduct inferential statistical tests that provide p-values, and they often conclude that findings are important solely because the p-value is found to be "statistically significant" (i.e., $p < 0.05$). Interpretation of the pattern of findings (e.g., treatment group performs better than the control group) then proceeds, and researchers make conclusions and recommendations based on such analysis simply because p was less than 0.05. Recent literature reflects a different approach—while statistical significance is desired, the size of the detected effect (e.g., the difference in the means for the control vs. treatment group; the size of a correlation coefficient; the odds ratio) is what many believe should actually be interpreted. In this approach, the question to be asked (and answered) is: *Is the effect size found sufficiently large to have clinical or practical importance, irrespective of statistical significance*? With relatively large samples, it is common to find statistically significant effects that have little clinical importance (i.e., the treatment effect is small or not worth the treatment costs or adverse effects that occur or is not large enough to have much practical benefit to patients or enough impact to justify the cost of treatments or the burden of adverse effects). Thus, it is critical to determine the *minimum clinically important difference* (MCID) a priori before study conduct and then to interpret study outcomes in view of the MCID. Once statistical significance is demonstrated, then interpretation of outcomes should only be framed by whether the treatment effect is worthwhile in terms of symptom reduction, cost of treatment, and adverse effects [3]. These assessments will also offer information that relates to the best available alternative treatments already identified as efficacious and effective (e.g., the evidence-based standard of care).

Sixth, researchers often report outcomes with insufficient details about how the study outcomes were produced because journals severely limit space allocated to author reports. That is, details from the study protocol are not included in the article, which are necessary to enable a reader to properly evaluate the validity or meaning of study outcomes or to attempt to replicate the original outcomes. In the past decade, increasing efforts have been made to *provide full protocols to those who evaluate studies* (e.g., proposals to post study protocols on accessible online databases), but the general access to study protocols remains quite low. How a treatment was actually implemented may greatly influence the size of the treatment effect and how any detected treatment effect (i.e., outcome) is interpreted. Without access to protocol details, readers of reports of study outcomes are usually faced with simply accepting the results on face value. This may lead to other researchers' efforts to replicate findings by using a protocol that is inconsistent with the original protocol, perhaps thus leading to failures to replicate the original results and in turn producing contradictory findings in the literature. This situation confuses other researchers, practitioners, and the public and greatly slows scientific and clinical progress.

Key Concepts

- *Efficacy* refers to the ability of a treatment to cause a beneficial effect. In health research efficacy is ideally demonstrated with a well-controlled and unconfounded randomized clinical trial. The intervention tested could involve a drug, a medical device, a surgical procedure, a physical therapy, behavioral therapy, or a public health treatment. Efficacy is demonstrated by showing that the experimental intervention or treatment produces a statistically significantly greater benefit than a control treatment. Whether the demonstrated effect has clinical significance is then shown by indicating that the size of effect statistically detected is sufficiently large and likely to have practical levels of benefit in terms of improvement in patient condition, cost, reduction in side effects, and other practical factors. That is, statistically efficacious effects may well be outweighed by excessive cost, serious side effects, or other practical problems.

- *Effectiveness* refers to the ability of a treatment placed into actual practice environments to have beneficial effects on patients. Many treatments with demonstrated efficacy in practice do not show effectiveness because many factors operating in natural environments may detract from the direct effect of a treatment. For example, some treatments in practice may have such low rates of compliance among patients that they do not in the long run show sufficient degrees of benefit. Treatments with clearly demonstrated efficacy in highly controlled and artificial clinical trial settings may not show effectiveness under normal practice conditions.

- *Translational Research* refers to studies of how to transform study findings from controlled research environments into real-world practice environments. Currently, translational research is categorized as T1, T2, or T3 types. T1 translation takes a research finding made in a laboratory (often called "the bench") to a new treatment

(continued)

(continued)

tested in clinical (usually called "the bedside") studies. In contrast, T2 translation takes results from clinical studies to everyday clinical practice and health decision-making settings. Finally, T3 translation integrates evidence-based treatment guidelines into actual healthcare practice through delivery and dissemination.

- *Systematic reviews* examine the mechanisms underlying a phenomenon and usually focus on intervention, diagnosis, or prognosis in biomedical fields. Systematic reviews can help practitioners and researchers to be kept well-informed about outcomes in the medical literature by summarizing large bodies of evidence and helping to explain differences among studies dealing with the same question. A systematic review applies scientific strategies in ways that limit bias to the assembly, critical appraisal, and synthesis of all relevant studies that address a specific research question. A meta-analysis is a specific type of systematic review that uses statistical methods to combine and summarize the results of several primary studies that utilized conceptually similar independent and dependent variables.

Seventh, no single study proves anything in science. *Replication of findings is essential* to establish confidence in the validity of study outcomes. Efforts to replicate findings commonly fail in biomedical science—still, such replication failures are not definitive because there are many reasons that studies may fail, only one of which is that the findings are not real. One of the reasons I have emphasized in this chapter—studies are often methodologically weak or flawed. It may take several replication efforts to isolate the reasons that different versions of the same study produce different outcomes. Are there differences in study designs, conduct, sample sizes, or analysis of studies with positive outcomes vs. those with null or negative outcomes? In addition, failures to replicate previous findings are less likely to be published than positive outcomes, and this bias distorts the understanding of phenomenon that can be gained from simply reading the published literature. Replicated study results increase our confidence that study outcomes are valid.

Assessing Outcomes Reported in the Literature. It is unlikely that all relevant articles in an area lead clearly to the same conclusion. How do you assess the whole picture, which probably includes some conflicting results, at least in terms of effects sizes, and certainly includes studies that have varying characteristics and methods, even if they have the same general objective?

Three basic types of reviews can be found. *Narrative reviews* critically appraise and summarize primary literature on a common topic area, but they do not set specific criteria for selecting literature to be included or for specific review protocol. A narrative review draws together major arguments in a field of research. Narrative reviews today only should be conducted on topics that do not lend themselves to systematic reviews. Narrative reviews used to be the most common review in the literature, and it was not unusual for different reviewers to publish rather different assessments of the literature only a decade or two ago. Today, the accepted standard is for a *systematic review* to examine the mechanisms underlying a phenomenon and usually focus on intervention, diagnosis, or prognosis in biomedical fields. Systematic reviews help practitioners and researchers to keep abreast of the medical literature by summarizing large bodies of evidence and helping to explain differences among studies dealing with the same question. A systematic review applies scientific strategies in ways that limit bias to the assembly, critical appraisal, and synthesis of all relevant studies that address a specific research question [4, 5]. A *meta-analysis* is a specific type of systematic review that uses statistical methods to combine and summarize the results of several primary studies that share similar independent or predictor variables and outcome variables. A meta-analysis is very useful when a set of studies on a phenomenon show different effect sizes or have two sets of studies, one set showing one effect and the other the more or less opposite effect.

Readers also consult textbooks and other scholarly books to gain an overview of the phenomenon of interest. Textbooks have limitations that are different than those in the primary literature—textbooks are at least 2–4 years behind the literature, they tend to make conservative conclusions that do not reflect emerging literature at the time they are published, and they certainly make global pronouncements that may be far less useful than more specific primary articles in particular contexts.

The final decision about the value of a study or set of studies rests with the reader. I have encouraged readers to not be intimidated by the power of the printed word, especially if it is found in prestigious journals, to do the best work possible in one's academic role. Each reader must make an independent assessment.

Words to the Wise

As you evaluate research studies and their outcomes, ask and answer the following questions:

- Having appraised (rather than merely read) an article, do you generally believe the study results and conclusions? If not, what are your reasons for disbelief?
- What plausible alternative interpretations exist for the reported study outcomes?
- What novel and nontrivial contributions to the literature do the study results make?
- Do you understand how the study results fit with other published work and knowledge?
- How might any study weaknesses be remedied (e.g., research design, sampling, procedures, statistical analysis, reporting) if someone were to undertake the study again?
- How might a new study be designed in a way to *extend* the findings of a published study?

Ask Your Mentor or Colleagues

- How can I gain a greater understanding of the concept of validity of measures and outcomes?
- How do we search for systematic reviews, especially Cochrane reviews? For other sources of systematic reviews?

(continued)

(continued)
- Do I have skills and knowledge regarding research design, conduct, analysis, and reporting sufficient to enable your competent evaluation of complex research? Do I need to consider additional formal training or independent study with mentors to enhance these skills?

References

1. Woolf SH. The meaning of translational research and why it matters. J Am Med Assoc. 2008;299(2):211–3.
2. Sechrest L. Validity of measures is no simple matter. Health Res Edu Trust. 40(5)Part II:1584–604.
3. Ziliak ST, McCloskey DN. The cult of statistical significance: how the standard error costs us jobs, justice, and lives. Ann Arbor, MI: University of Michigan Press.
4. Liberati A, Altman DG, Tetzlaff J, Mulrow C, Goetzsche PC, et al. The PRISMA Statement for reporting systematic reviews and meta-analyses of studies that evaluate health care interventions: explanation and elaboration. PLoS Med. 2009;6(7):e1000100.
5. Moher D, Liberati A, Tetzlaff J, Altman DG. The PRISMA Group preferred reporting items for systematic reviews and meta-analyses. PLoS Med. 2009;6(7):e1000097.

Further Reading

Gelbach SH. Interpreting the medical literature, 5th ed. New York: McGraw-Hill; 2006.
Guyatt G, Rennie D, Meade M, Cook D. Users' guides to the medical literature: a manual for evidence-based clinical practice, 2nd ed. New York: McGraw-Hill; 2008.
Piantadosi S. Clinical trials: a methodologic perspective, 2nd ed. New York: Wiley; 2005.
Stone J. Conducting clinical research: a practical guide for physicians, nurses, study coordinators, and investigators. Cumberland, MD: Mountainside Maryland Press; 2010.
Wang D, Bukai A. Clinical trials—a practical guide to design, analysis, and reporting. London: Remedica Publishing; 2006.

How to Maintain Excellent Clinical Documentation

14

Justin A. Birnbaum

Clinical documentation and navigation of the medical record are part of every practitioner's daily activities. This documentation and the associated medical recordkeeping requirements are central to the provision of excellent clinical care. At times, documentation tasks may be perceived as a burden. In reality, however, they are a necessary and extremely useful component of clinical practice.

Multiple essential functions are served by the medical record. These functions include communication, quality measures, compliance, research, and medicolegal coverage, all of which are described further in the subsequent text.

Communication. Medical records serve as the basis for communication between health care professionals. This documentation provides a reliable reference for clinicians regarding their thought process over time. It acquaints clinicians of the evolution of care provided and the logic associated with medical decisions. It informs about diagnostic formulations and uncertainties, interventions, outcomes, and complications. These benefits are achieved with documentation that is accurate, timely, complete, and concise.

J.A. Birnbaum, M.D. (✉)
Department of Psychiatry and Behavioral Sciences, Stanford University, 401 Quarry Rd MC 5723, Stanford, CA, USA
e-mail: justin.birnbaum@stanford.edu

© Springer International Publishing Switzerland 2016
L.W. Roberts (ed.), *The Clinician Educator Guidebook*,
DOI 10.1007/978-3-319-27980-0_14

Quality Measures. The medical record is increasingly accessed to measure achievement of goals set to improve patient care. The goals may be set by external regulatory bodies, such as the Joint Commission for Hospital Accreditation or Centers for Medicare and Medicaid Services (CMS), or developed by a particular institution or department. These measures are often viewed as aggregate data for an institution but also can be directed toward the practice pattern of individual clinicians. The efforts aim to improve patient care via use of the medical record, in part by assisting clinicians to identify areas of potential improvement in clinical practice and monitor these over time to determine if goals are being met. Additionally, if questions arise as to standards of care being met by an individual clinician in specific instances, the medical record is essential in the review of such circumstances.

Compliance. The medical record is the basis through which individuals or institutions validate each patient care interaction as it relates to the extent of care provided. This, in turn, is directly related to billing and reimbursement. The clinical documentation should reflect the complexity of care provided and/or time involved in care, and this should be reflected in the billing request. In order for compliance standards to be met, it is necessary for clinicians to have an adequate understanding of appropriate documentation and coding guidelines. This is a challenge.

Research. Data available through the medical record are a resource for healthcare researchers. Accurate, accessible clinical data may provide valuable information and significantly influence evidence-based practice. With the advent of the electronic medical/health record, this source of research data will likely continue to expand greatly.

Medical/Legal. The medical record serves as the official documentation of care provision in circumstances in which legal matters become entwined with clinical care, such as questions regarding informed consent for medical treatments or standards of medical practice being met. Clear and complete documentation is key in these circumstances. Incomplete records may be as detrimental as inaccurate records in legal proceedings.

The Electronic Medical Record

In academic centers, the medical/health record is often an amalgam of information that may include descriptive data that are written, typed, or dictated by clinicians, laboratory results, radiologic images, photographs or drawings, demographic data, self-report forms completed by patients, written communications from families, insurance carrier communications, pharmacy records, and a variety of other contents. Each institution has its own processes to manage its medical records, and it is essential to understand how the institution in which you work manages this information. Endless options exist in regard to how medical information is obtained, stored, and accessed. Important first steps to help one understand his or her institution's system are knowing the following:

1. Who is responsible for the various data entries (including updating of data)—clinicians and support staff?
2. Where the information is stored—electronic and hard copies?
3. How to most effectively enter and access the stored information? This may require initial training and intermittent training updates (often time well spent).

When becoming familiar with the methods that a particular institution utilizes to organize and manage its medical records, one will likely have personal preferences regarding the process. While it is fair to advocate for one's individual preferences, this is often limited by the need for, and benefits of, standardization of these methods. It will be useful to recall that most systems have been built to meet the varied purposes the medical documentation serves.

Paper-based records have been the standard for medical record-keeping and in most settings are currently being replaced, or already have been replaced, by electronic, computer-based systems. This Electronic Medical Record (EMR) will eventually replace the paper with an electronic record that maintains the elements of the traditional paper-based method and, it is believed, will eventually provide significant additional capabilities and benefits:

- Computerized access to information has the potential to streamline the clinician's workflow.

- Improved access to accurate clinical information and data will improve clinical care by improving clinical decision-making and reducing risks.
- Improved communication between patients and clinicians.
- Increased patient awareness and involvement in care.
- Improved evidence-based decision support by providing prompts and reminders to clinicians.
- Enhanced data collection for research and quality management processes.
- Reduced health care costs by increased integration of care (e.g., reduced duplication of tests, reduced delays in treatment).
- Minimized reimbursement discrepancies as documentation and billing processes are coupled.

The transition to use of the EMR has been slow and is not without its challenges. Some items worth considering are these:

- The transfer of data (historic and current) from hard copy to the EMR is arduous and accuracy is essential. Be informed about the systems in place to ensure that the EMR data are accurate and complete.
- Updating data is as important as initial data entry. Who is responsible for updating EMR data?
- Systems and methods to minimize information overload are needed. Both institutions and individuals should design strategies to make the EMR complete, but concise. For example, "Copying Forward" of electronic documentation has utility if used appropriately, but may result in a burdensome excess of information if inappropriately used.
- Patient access to clinical information carries benefits but requires thoughtful processes to manage patient responses. Be aware of these processes and ask for assistance if unclear.
- Clinical templates for documentation are effective tools if designed correctly. Ask about redesign if these templates do not fit your clinical practice.
- Standardized or templated clinical documentation may not be sufficient in the clinical setting where the narrative description is central to clinical practice.

Basics of Excellent Clinical Documentation Entry

The clinical documentation provided by a professional is a testament to the care provided to a patient and, as such, should be thoughtfully entered into the medical record. Basic, but important, considerations are noted below.

- Be accurate and honest, including uncertainties.
- Be clear and describe your thought process in clinical decision making.
- Be complete and concise.
- Minimize duplication.
- Identify sources of information.
- Include contacts with family.
- Be timely with entries—same day whenever possible.
- Maintain transparency when correcting errors or making late entries in record.
- Avoid use of idiosyncratic abbreviations.
- Include informed consent.

Privacy and Clinical Documentation

Maintaining confidentiality and privacy of the medical record has been an expectation for many years and increasing regulatory requirements have been implemented over the last few decades. The US Department of Health and Human Services (HHS) issued the Privacy Rule to implement the requirement of the Health Insurance Portability and Accountability Act of 1996 (HIPAA). Compliance with the Privacy Rule standards was expected by, and initiated in, April 2003. The Privacy Rule standards address the use and disclosure of individuals' health information.

In the era of the EMR, maintaining excellent documentation means, in part, complying with privacy standards in an evolving and increasingly complex environment. Some suggestions:

- Maintain confidentiality of passwords and update them as required.
- Do not transfer patient data to unsecure sites.

- If any patient data are viewable via "smart-phone" connections, make sure that the phone is pass-code protected.
- Use electronic communications (e.g., e-mail) containing any patient information only as approved by the institution.
- Use confidentiality statements when using electronic communications.
- Log off computer access when leaving any work station.
- Do not download any documentation containing patient data to a personal computer.
- If a personal computer has remote access to patient data, make sure that the access is closed when leaving the computer unattended.
- When viewing electronic information on a monitor, make sure that others cannot view the screen.
- Medical records should not be left in an unlocked room or be left unattended.
- Report a breach or potential breach of confidentiality immediately.

Compliance, Clinical Documentation, and Financial Considerations

Compliance as it relates to clinicians in practice is a term that refers to the extent to which the clinical care provided, and the associated documentation of that care, is in accordance with the service/procedure code applied to that provision of care. The Physicians' Current Procedural Terminology (CPT) is published annually by the American Medical Association (AMA). It is a systematic listing and coding of procedures and services performed by physicians and other healthcare professionals. A five-digit code is provided for each procedure or service. The intent of the CPT codes is to simplify the reporting of medical services. The desire is for CPT codes to be used appropriately and accurately so as to reflect the true level of care provided (as reflected in the clinical documentation). If this is achieved, the clinical encounter is deemed "within compliance."

The ability to remain "in compliance" when providing clinical care, documenting this care, and then selecting the appropriate CPT code is directly correlated with the clinician's awareness and memory around CPT codes. It is not surprising that many clinicians do not fully remember the criteria expected to fulfill each CPT code that they might utilize when providing care to patients. This may result in the use of CPT codes that "under-code" or "over-code" the patient care interaction. It is important to make efforts to ensure that clinicians are not consistently "under-coding" or "over-coding" for services/procedures as this may have significant financial implications and/or result in regulatory penalties. Many institutions have developed compliance departments to assist with this matter, and provide reference cards for clinicians' use.

Three suggestions:

1. Limit the number of CPT codes you utilize. Be familiar with the criteria for a few CPT codes and investigate other codes when necessary.
2. Avoid consistently "under-coding" or "over-coding."
3. Ask for assistance from the Compliance Department when starting practice and when difficulties arise.

CPT codes are associated with certain monetary values in financial reimbursement. Accurate use of CPT codes is important for appropriate billing of services for both the individual clinician and the institution. Frequently, a clinician's salary is covered by an institution based upon financial billing targets, or determined by the institution based upon financial billings. The CPT codes submitted for reimbursement by the clinician are significant determinants in meeting financial billing expectations.

Another method of measuring clinical work productivity is based on work relative value units (wRVUs). Each CPT code has an associated wRVU that assigns a numeric reimbursement value. The clinical documentation required for CPT code and wRVU pairs is identical. Whether it be CPT code (and associated financial billings) or wRVU driven, clinicians working in an environment that has set clinical productivity based on either of these measures are wise to strategize about achieving their productivity target.

Consider the following:

- Have a clear understanding of clinical work productivity targets.
- Discuss any question or concerns about targets with a supervisor early in the fiscal year.
- Request monthly reports to ensure that productivity is on track.
- Productivity will increase over time as one's practice is established.
- Take into account the effect of anticipated leaves of absence.
- Anticipate fluctuations in month-to-month productivity.
- Discuss in a timely manner any anticipated changes in expected clinical productivity due to restructuring of employment responsibilities (e.g., changes in research funding or administrative responsibilities) with a supervisor/administrator.
- Request a meeting with compliance administrators if available.

Words to the Wise
- Be accurate and honest, including uncertainties.
- Be timely with entries—same day whenever possible.
- Be aware that productivity will increase over time.

Ask Your Mentor or Colleagues
- Given the significance of matching clinical care and its associated documentation with appropriate CPT codes, when might it be possible to use the EMR to automatically generate appropriate CPT coding?
- With the increase of patient accessibility to the medical record, do you have suggestions for managing this?
- How do I most directly get help for questions about the EMR?

How to Avoid Medicolegal Problems

15

Liliana Kalogjera Barry

> *Patients want physicians to be sensitive and caring as only humans can be, but they also want physicians to perform in the consistent and controlled manner of machines [1].*

Fear of medical malpractice litigation is a common concern among both novice and seasoned physicians, and the quotation above captures the pressure many may feel to practice in a manner that achieves perfection in both the humanistic and technical aspects of medicine. It is highly likely, if not inevitable, that a physician who practices for a significant amount of time will eventually commit some sort of error or participate in a case involving an unfortunate outcome. However, there are ways for a physician to avoid medicolegal problems in the first place and strategies for dealing with the medicolegal problems that occur in a manner that minimizes risk while honoring the physician's ethical and other professional obligations.

L.K. Barry, M.D. (✉)
Department of Psychiatry and Behavioral Medicine, Medical College of Wisconsin, 8701 Watertown Plank Road, Milwaukee, WI, USA
e-mail: lilianakalogjera@gmail.com

© Springer International Publishing Switzerland 2016
L.W. Roberts (ed.), *The Clinician Educator Guidebook*,
DOI 10.1007/978-3-319-27980-0_15

The Reality of Medical Malpractice Litigation

An important aspect to avoiding medical legal problems is a basic understanding of the landscape of medical malpractice litigation in the United States. How often do patients sue their physicians? How often do physicians lose such lawsuits? What are some of the predictive factors associated with the initiation of a medical malpractice lawsuit? These are just some of the many relevant questions physicians may have.

The following data provide context for the legal issues physicians may face:

- A landmark 1999 study by the Institute of Medicine found that as many as 98,000 deaths annually in US hospitals are attributable to preventable medical errors [2].
- Despite the high rate of medical error, there is a mismatch between medical error and medical malpractice suits: most patients who are injured by medical malpractice do not file lawsuits, and there are many plaintiffs in medical malpractice cases who were not victims of negligence [3].
- The American Medical Association's 2007–2008 Physician Practice Information Survey found that while a physician's risk of being sued in a given year is relatively low, 5 %, 61 % of physicians 55 years old or older have been sued during the course of their careers [4].
- The AMA study also determined that risk of being sued varies by specialty, estimating that as few as 22.2 % of psychiatrists and as many as 69.2 % of surgeons and obstetricians/gynecologists have been sued [4].
- A study by Studdert et al. [5] concluded that, despite the risk of being sued, generalizations that the US medical malpractice system is "stricken with frivolous litigation" are overblown; most claims that involve errors do not result in payment.
- Feld and Moses estimate that approximately 80 % of physicians prevail in a medical malpractice suit and cite another landmark study by Harvard University, which examined medical malpractice claims in New York and concluded that there are fewer lawsuits than incidents of medical negligence [6].

- A physician's risk of being sued appears stable over time and related to "patients' dissatisfaction with their physicians' ability to establish rapport, provide access, administer care and treatment consistent with expectations and communicate effectively" [7].
- Physician concerns about being sued result in changes in clinical practice in order to avoid liability, also known as "defensive medicine" [8].

As a whole, the data suggest that although a physician's risk of being sued for malpractice is real, it is also nuanced. There are predictive clues of litigation risk and, thus, strategies physicians can take to avoid being sued.

The following strategies for physicians represent attainable means to prevent litigation: (1) be aware of clinical expectations, (2) communicate and document well, (3) consider disclosure, (4) remember ethical considerations, and (5) utilize institutional resources. Although this chapter focuses on avoiding "litigation," the same strategies are applicable for avoiding less formal types of medicolegal issues, e.g., patient complaints, credentialing and privileging problems, and reporting to the state licensing board and National Practitioner Data Bank.

Strategy 1: Be Aware of Clinical Expectations

An important aspect of avoiding litigation is to "concentrate on good medicine without obsessing about the risk of legal liability" [8]. "Good medicine" involves both meeting the standard of care and avoiding unwarranted defensive medicine.

When facing a lawsuit for medical negligence, the law holds a physician with a duty to a particular patient to the "standard of care," which consists of "that medical care that would be provided by a reasonable physician in the same or similar circumstances" [9]. In addition to proving that a physician breached the standard of care, a plaintiff must also establish that he or she was harmed and that the harm was caused by the deviation from the standard of care [9].

Courts typically rely on expert testimony to establish whether the physician acted reasonably under the circumstances. Exceptions to this practice occur when the negligence was so obvious that "the thing speaks for itself," *res ipsa loquitor*, e.g., a surgery performed on the wrong side of the body or a surgery resulting in a retained instrument [10]. Clinical practice guidelines, medical literature, and other forms of evidence-based medicine may also be relevant for establishing the standard of care, and their use in litigation appears to be growing, albeit with some controversy [11]. Regardless of the formal use of clinical practice guidelines in litigation, however, staying current on the developments within one's specialty helps to ensure that a physician is aware of the standard of care, which may evolve over time.

In addition to meeting the standard of care, physicians should avoid overcompensating for liability concerns by practicing unwarranted defensive medicine, medicine which aims primarily to avoid lawsuit as opposed to benefitting patients. Examples include ordering extra tests, procedures, and referrals [3]. Unwarranted defensive medicine is problematic both pragmatically and ethically. Defensive medicine may expose physicians to potential liability if it is not clinically indicated, and it raises ethical concerns such as the potential conflict of interest between the physician's fiduciary duty to the patient and personal interest in avoiding litigation, which is discussed in greater detail below.

Strategy 2: Communicate and Document Well

Communication and documentation, a written form of communication, are critical aspects of litigation prevention.

Numerous studies have found that poor communication, rather than negligence, is the primary reason people sue [12]. Hickson et al. examined patient complaints and malpractice risk and found that, consistent with previously published studies, "[p]atients who saw physicians with the highest numbers of lawsuits were more likely to complain that their physicians would not listen or return telephone calls, were rude and did not show respect," and those who sued their physicians expressed similar concerns [7]. Another study by Vincent et al. found that, in addition to the initial injury, "insensitive handling and poor communication after the original incident" led to litigation [13]. May and Aulisio cited one study identifying communication problems generally as the driving factor in over 80 % of medical malpractice cases, and others that found a link between specific communication problems, e.g., concerns about cover-ups or the desire for revenge, and lawsuits [14].

Physicians can practice good communication with patients by communicating "in an honest, open, empathetic manner" [8]. This includes listening to patients, following up with patients, and treating patients respectfully and with sensitivity to their particular situation. It also includes incorporating a meaningful informed consent process in the course of each patient's care. When unfortunate outcomes arise, good communication includes appropriate disclosure, as discussed below. It both reduces liability exposure and is consistent with the ethical standards set forth by the American Medical Association and the American College of Physicians [8].

Communication with other health care providers and/or the treatment team is also of critical importance and may help to prevent systems errors or situations when a patient "falls through the cracks." Avoidance of systems errors is particularly important given the fact that the 1999 Institute of Medicine Report concluded that most medical errors are due to flawed systems and processes and not individual negligence [2]. Williams provides the following examples of such systems failures: "[c]ulture reports, other laboratory and pathology reports, and radiology reports not being timely seen by or communicated by the ordering physician;" "[r]eferrals or consults ordered, but not made or obtained;" "[i]mportant laboratory results or other information to be discussed with the patient at the next appointment, but the patient cancels or no-shows and the important information is not communicated to the patient;" "[w]rong medication administered;" "[m]edication allergies not appreciated or overlooked;" and "[c]ritical medical history missed which exists in prior records in the same facility" [15]. Physicians can help to prevent systems errors by ensuring that all relevant information is transmitted to other providers during transitions in care such as shift changes and other time periods when the risk of lapses in care may increase.

In addition to preventing systems errors, communication with other physicians may also help to provide justification for a physician's actions. For example, a physician may wish to obtain a consult for a difficult or unusual case or one calling for treatment other than what is typical [16]. Such justification may prove useful in the event medicolegal problems arise for the physician in the future.

Documentation serves the dual functions of communicating and providing proof of communication, hence the common catch-phrase among risk management and legal professionals that "if it's not documented, it didn't happen." Among providers, the medical record is meant to transmit all pertinent information about a patient's status, history, and treatment plan and is, thus, a vital component of patient safety. If potential litigation arises, the medical record may also prove useful in a physician's defense by providing evidence of discussions between the physician and patient and insight into the rationale behind treatment decisions, which may be particularly valuable in a case involving a deviation from a clinical practice guideline [16]. The litigation of a single medical malpractice matter can take many years, and good documentation is crucial to ensure that favorable evidence is preserved.

Strategy 3: Consider Disclosure

Disclosure of medical errors and adverse outcomes is closely related to good communication. In the event of a medical error or adverse outcome, a physician should consult with the institution's risk management professionals and consider whether and how to disclose the error or outcome to the patient.

Contrary to what some may expect, existing data support disclosure as a means for reducing litigation risk. Two frequently cited examples include a study involving the US Department of Veterans Affairs (VA) Medical Center in Lexington, Kentucky and one at the University of Michigan Health System.

Following two losses in medical malpractice cases that totaled over $1.5 million, the VA Medical Center in Lexington adopted a humanistic approach to risk management that included proactively identifying medical errors and accidents and, following investigation of the facts, fully disclosing the incidents to patients and/or their next of kin, providing the patient or next of kin with opportunity to file a claim, and attempting to settle any corresponding claims in a timely, fair manner [17]. The VA subsequently adopted a policy of full disclosure of adverse events for all of its facilities, and the results appear promising. For example, from 1990 through 1996, the average payment on a tort claim by the Lexington VA Medical Center was only $15,622, and the average private sector judgment for medical malpractice cases is approximately double that for the VA system ($1,484,000 versus $720,000) [17].

Similarly, the University of Michigan Health System began implementing a program of full disclosure and compensation of medical errors in 2001 [18]. Since implementation of the program, the University of Michigan has seen a decrease in the number of claims, liability costs, and length of time to resolve the claims [18].

These and other studies appear to have prompted legal efforts to promote disclosure of medical errors at the federal and state level. In 2005, then Senators Hillary Rodham Clinton and Barack Obama proposed the National Medical Error Disclosure and Compensation (MEDiC) Bill (S. 1784) [19]. Although the MEDiC Bill did not become law, it represented a national-level effort to promote full disclosure of medical error, timely and fair compensation for such errors, and subsequent patient safety efforts to prevent recurrence [12, 19]. A 2008 study by McDonnell and Guenther found that 36 states have adopted apology laws to protect disclosure of medical errors, with 28 of the states barring the use of expressions of sympathy, regret, and condolence against the physician in subsequent litigation [19]. Other states have laws requiring disclosure of medical errors involving adverse outcomes and prohibiting such disclosures from serving as evidence of fault in malpractice litigation [19]. Similarly, since 2001, the Joint Commission has required disclosure of care that caused harm [20].

Due to the variation in laws regarding disclosure of medical errors and institution-specific policies, a physician should check with the facility's risk management professionals for advice on how to proceed if the need for disclosure arises. Assuming that disclosure is warranted, the risk management professionals should also be able to provide guidance on how to disclose incidents. Woods describes the key elements as "recognition, regret, responsibility, remedy, and remaining engaged" [21]. The VA approach includes a face-to-face meeting, in which key staff provide the details of the case in a sensitive manner, communicate the facility and personnel's regret, describe any corrective action taken to prevent reoccurrence, and offer to answer questions and provide restitution, e.g., through corrective treatment or financial compensation [17]. Additional tips include empathizing with the patient and family, communicating the bad news in an immediate and direct manner, expressing sorrow for the person's loss, and documenting the disclosure in the chart [1]. Note that while disclosure should always be complete and truthful, some disclosure approaches advocate framing the apology in a manner that conveys regret for what happened as opposed to apologizing for the physicians' actions [1]. In addition, whether disclosing an error or making a medical record entry, physicians should generally focus on the clinical facts and avoid making legal conclusions, such as statements that treatment was "negligent" or "substandard."

Strategy 4: Remember Ethical Concerns

Although a physician should always be mindful of the ethical obligations that arise with the practice of medicine, this awareness is particularly important when facing medicolegal issues, due to the increased potential for conflicts of interest. A physician may face many varying ethical or contractual obligations including those to patients, employers, and medical malpractice insurance carriers and other legal obligations (e.g., state-based duties to report medical errors). These obligations may compete with each other, for example, when the physician's employer advises that the physician take a course of action that is not in the patient's best interest, as would be the case if an employer advocated less than full disclosure of a medical error. The obligations may also present ethical challenges to the physician if his/her personal interests are distinct, for example, when disclosure of an adverse event may be ethically warranted but the physician feels pressure not to disclose due to personal fears of litigation and potential reporting to the state licensing board and National Practitioner Data Bank.

Despite these competing pressures, the physician's primary duty remains to the patient, as the doctor-patient relationship is fiduciary in nature, i.e., based on trust. As mandated in the Hippocratic Oath, patients trust their physicians to "do no harm," a concept known as "nonmaleficence," [22] along with the converse principle of doing good for the patient, "beneficence," which some see as the primary imperative of medicine [23]. In the event of an error or unfortunate event, the fiduciary nature of the doctor-patient relationship obligates the physician to be honest with the patient, an obligation that Woods has characterized as an extension of the informed consent process or "ongoing informed consent" [21].

The American Medical Association's Code of Medical Ethics explicitly addresses the ethical obligations of physicians faced with potential disclosure issues at Opinion 8.12, Patient Information, which states the following:

> It is a fundamental ethical requirement that a physician should at all times deal honestly and openly with patients. Patients have a right to know their past and present medical status and to be free of any mistaken beliefs concerning their conditions. Situations occasionally occur in which a patient suffers significant medical complications that may have resulted from the physician's mistake or judgment. In these situations, the physician is ethically required to inform the patient of all the facts necessary to ensure understanding of what has occurred. Only through full disclosure is a patient able to make informed decisions regarding future medical care …

Concern regarding legal liability which might result following truthful disclosure should not affect the physician's honesty with a patient [24].

Closely related is the AMA Code of Ethics Opinion 8.03, Conflict of Interest: Guidelines, which states the following:

> Under no circumstances may physicians place their own financial interests above the welfare of their patients. The primary objective of the medical profession is to render service to humanity; reward or financial gain is a subordinate consideration. For a physician to unnecessarily hospitalize a patient, prescribe a drug, or conduct diagnostic tests for the physician's financial benefit is unethical. If a conflict develops between the physician's financial interest and the physician's responsibilities to the patient, the conflict must be resolved to the patient's benefit [24].

A physician who practices unwarranted defensive medicine risks violating Opinion 8.03 if he/she orders unnecessary tests or treatment for purposes of avoiding litigation and its associated costs.

Thus, when faced with a medicolegal issue, a physician is ethically obligated to honor the primacy and fiduciary nature of the doctor-patient relationship by placing the best interests of the patient before any competing interests and engaging in complete, honest disclosure.

Strategy 5: Utilize Institutional Resources

Perhaps one of the biggest mistakes a physician can make in dealing with a medicolegal issue is to face it alone. Many institutional resources are available to prevent medicolegal issues and address existing ones. Such resources can help to minimize litigation risk and provide support to the physician facing the stress and other challenges associated with a medicolegal issue. As discussed above, good starting points include the institution's risk management professionals. These individuals have the necessary expertise to investigate the facts and coordinate an appropriate response, and they are knowledgeable about applicable law, institutional policy, and other requirements such as those set by the Joint Commission and state licensing boards. Physicians may also benefit from the less formal counsel and support offered by supervisors and peers. The institutional ethics committees may serve as another valuable resource; although not typically tasked with a risk management function, such committees can help to clarify clinical and ethical issues, identify stakeholders and decision makers, define legal and ethical boundaries, and resolve conflicts.

When indicated, e.g., institutional resources so advise or it appears that the physician's interests may diverge from the institution's and litigation is foreseeable, a physician should consider obtaining personal legal counsel and inform the physician's professional liability carrier [1].

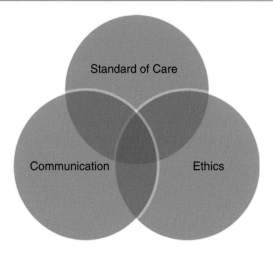

Fig. 15.1   Best practices model for avoiding medicolegal problems

Conclusion

In conclusion, "[t]he skilled and humane practice of medicine turns out to be the best form of risk management" [8]. When physicians practice good medicine, i.e., medicine that meets or exceeds the clinical standard of care, in an ethical manner and communicate well, they prevent medicolegal issues. See Fig. 15.1. However, even the best physicians may face legal scrutiny at some point. By continuing to adhere to professional ethical standards and communicating with patients, e.g., through appropriate disclosure of medical errors, physicians can minimize both patient harm and their personal liability exposure.

Words to the Wise
- Focus on practicing good, ethical medicine.
- Keep current on evolving clinical standards in your field.
- Maintain good communication with patients and other health care providers; documentation is the best proof of this.
- Seek help when facing a medicolegal issue.
- Disclose medical errors when appropriate.

Ask Your Mentor or Colleagues
- What resources does my institution offer for dealing with medicolegal problems, both preventatively and in response to litigation?
- What specific areas of my clinical practice are ripe for potential medicolegal problems?
- How can I improve the systems issues related to my clinical practice?
- What policies does my institution have regarding disclosure of medical errors and/or adverse events?

References

1. Charles SC, Frisch PR. A physician's guide: adverse events, stress and litigation. New York: Oxford University Press; 2005.
2. Kohn LT, Corrigan JM, Donaldson MS, editors. To err is human: building a safer health system. Washington, DC: National Academy Press; 2000.
3. Schoenbaum SC, Bovbjerg RR. Malpractice reform must include steps to prevent medical injury. Ann Intern Med. 2004;140:51–3.
4. Kane CT. Medical claim frequency: a 2007–2008 snapshot of physicians. Chicago, IL: American Medical Association; 2010.
5. Studdert DM, et al. Claims, errors, and compensation payments in medical malpractice litigation. N Engl J Med. 2006;354:2024–33.
6. Feld AD, Moses RE. Most doctors win: what to do if sued for medical malpractice. Am J Gastroenterol. 2009;104:1346–51.
7. Hickson GB, et al. Patient complaints and malpractice risk. JAMA. 2002;287:2951–7.
8. Forster HJ, Schwartz J, DeRenzo E. Reducing legal risk by practicing patient-centered medicine. Arch Intern Med. 2002;162:1217–9.
9. Ryan M. Medical malpractice: a review of issues for providers. Hematol Oncol Clin North Am. 2002;16: 1331–50.
10. Zane RD. The legal process. Emerg Med Clin North Am. 2009; 27:583–92.
11. Rosoff AJ. Evidence-based medicine and the law: the courts confront clinical practice guidelines. J Health Polit Policy Law. 2001;26(2): 327–68.
12. Clinton HR, Obama B. Making patient safety the centerpiece of medical liability reform. N Engl J Med. 2006;354(21):2205–10.

13. Vincent C, Young M, Phillips A. Why do people sue doctors? A study of patients and relatives taking legal action. Lancet. 1994;343:1609–13.
14. May T, Aulisio MP. Medical malpractice, mistake prevention, and compensation. Kennedy Inst Ethics J. 2001;11(2):135–46.
15. Williams DG. Practice patterns to decrease the risk of a malpractice suit. Clin Obstet Gynecol. 2008;51(4): 680–7.
16. Melonas JM, McNary AL. Taking action to avoid recurring risks in medical professional liability claims. Neurology. 2010;75 Suppl 1:S45–51.
17. Kraman SS, Hamm G. Risk management: extreme honesty may be the best policy. Ann Intern Med. 1999;131(12):963–7.
18. Kachalia A, et al. Liability claims and costs before and after implementation of a medical error disclosure program. Ann Intern Med. 2010; 153(4):213–21.
19. McDonnell WM, Guenther E. Narrative review: do state laws make it easier to say "I'm sorry?". Ann Intern Med. 2008;149(11):811–5.
20. Hellinger FJ, Encinosa WE. Review of reforms to our medical liability system. Rockville, MD: Agency for Healthcare Research and Quality; 2009.
21. Woods MS. Healing words: the power of apology in medicine. 2nd ed. Oakbrook Terrace, IL: Joint Commission Resources; 2007.
22. King NMP. Glossary of basic ethical concepts in health care and research. In: King NMP et al., editors. The social medicine reader. 2nd ed. Durham: Duke University Press; 2005. p. 161–8.
23. Churchill LR, King NMP, Schenk D. Ethics in medicine: an introduction to moral tools and traditions. In: King NMP et al., editors. The social medicine reader. 2nd ed. Durham: Duke University Press; 2005. p. 169–85.
24. AMA's Code of Medical Ethics. http://www.ama-assn.org/ama/pub/physician-resources/medical-ethics/code-medical-ethics.page. Accessed 7 Nov 2011

Further Reading

Sorry Works! Coalition Website. http://www.sorryworks.net/. Accessed 7 Nov 2011

How to Prepare the Best Possible Curriculum Vitae

16

Heather Kenna

The curriculum vitae (CV) is critical for early success in academic medicine. The CV should chronicle the academic physician's developing career in a way that provides a detailed overview of one's particular expertise and skillset in a clear and organized fashion. Over the course of a career in academic medicine, the CV can grow from a few pages in length to double-digit (and sometimes triple-digit) pages.

Learning to prepare a good CV early in one's career will aid the academic faculty member throughout his or her professional life, because the CV and its subspecies (e.g., bio sketch, resume, dossier) are vital to the scholar in academic medicine for achievement of institutional advancement and research funding [1, 2]. Some experts recommend maintaining two versions of the CV—one, a short summary of training and experiences; the other, a longer version with more detailed information about scholarly work. Because of the nature of the medical profession, in which the years of preparation are highly structured and generally comparable from institution to institution, a chronological format for the academic medicine CV is often preferred.

H. Kenna, M.A. (✉)
Department of Psychiatry and Behavioral Sciences, Stanford University,
401 Quarry Road, Stanford, CA, USA
e-mail: hkenna@stanford.edu

© Springer International Publishing Switzerland 2016   227
L.W. Roberts (ed.), *The Clinician Educator Guidebook*,
DOI 10.1007/978-3-319-27980-0_16

Despite its multiple purposes, the CV must be restructured or rewritten, or at least reviewed, for each purpose for which it is to be used. For example, if the academic physician is submitting an application for membership in a community organization, it might not be appropriate to include a lengthy list of publications in the CV, whereas it would be imperative to include this information in a CV submitted to obtain an academic position.

Commit to Keeping the CV Updated

For the early-career academic faculty member in medicine, the CV should be valued as a "living document" that is kept updated in a systematic, chronological manner. Although this may seem to be a daunting task, with effort and a bit of planning, one can develop a system to track CV data in a way that works well for individual schedules and lifestyles.

Find a way that works well for tracking data for the CV. Consider using a CV database, such as in Microsoft Excel or Endnote, to which publications, conference proceedings, lectures, honors and awards, committee work, and community service (among others) might be added in an ongoing fashion. Or use an old-fashioned box or accordion file to collect hard copy evidence of talks, papers, committees, teaching, and other academic activities. The key is to periodically review one's files to update the content of the CV. However this task is achieved, it will reward the academic physician with a blossoming textual history of one's work—a history that clearly communicates one's unique interests and expertise.

Consideration of CV Format

In academic medicine, the CV should summarize education and training in one's field, as well as one's scholarship, leadership, and other qualifications specific to the missions of academia (i.e., education, research, clinical service). CV length will vary depending on individual academic achievements (e.g., publications, conference proceedings, lectures, institutional and professional service).

Although the content in one's CV should follow an institution's suggested format and emphasize data related to the institution's mission and goals, the CV should generally always contain the following:

- Demographic and academic data: Name and contact information, academic and faculty rank and positions, education and training, board certifications, licensures (if applicable), and military service.
- Professional affiliations and leadership: Professional society memberships, including offices held and committee responsibilities.
- Faculty roles and activities: Typically includes research, education, clinical and community service, and local leadership roles.
- Scholarly representation and recognition: Bibliography (e.g., articles, book chapters, books), presentations at professional meetings, research grants and awards, manuscript review and editorial service, and grant review service.

Subheadings are helpful to organize the content of the CV and make it easy for reviewers. Presented in the appendix is a simple, sample CV formatted to reflect Professional Experience, Education, Credentials, Bibliography, Teaching and Mentoring, and Professional Organization Membership and Service. Other section subheadings may also be used, as needed, to reflect more unique categories of experience and/or expertise.

In preparing the CV, consider the mission goals of the institution for which it is geared. For example, is the institution strongly committed to community partnership? If so, the candidate might consider creating a special subsection in the CV to highlight specific work in this area (e.g., community lectures on disease X or syndrome Y, local volunteer service).

Be sure to check the CV formatting requirements specific to a particular institution. For example, some institutions require publications to be clustered and subtitled in a particular way, such as "Peer Reviewed" and "Non-Peer Reviewed" or "Invited", as opposed to a larger combined, chronological list of publications and other scholarly activities that may also include conference proceedings and lectures. Some institutions prefer that the physician's name be in bold within the bibliography to aid reviewers with respect to authorship order.

"Team Science" Annotations in the Bibliography

Authorship practices across disciplines in academic medicine follow a traditional pattern in which the first author listed is the primary author, and the last author listed is the senior author associated with the work [3]. There is a growing prevalence of collaborative "team science" scholarly work in academic medicine, which can create a challenge for reviewers (e.g., grant or academic committee members) to determine the nature of individual substantive contributions to middle-authored works listed in a CV (i.e., those not first- or senior-authored). As such, annotations are increasingly used in bibliographies to provide clarification. Annotations also allow the opportunity to *highlight* unique contributions across studies and collaborative work. This practice may be especially useful for early-career academic faculty members, who may have a greater proportion of middle-authored publications on their CVs and wish to highlight their work on a substantive paper in a high-impact journal. Annotation format and content may vary, but usually include a brief statement of one's role in a publication, such as involvement in the conception and design of a study, acquisition of data, statistical analysis and interpretation of data, and/or drafting of the manuscript. As one's career flourishes and publications increase in number, annotations may be reserved for use in more recent and/or higher impact papers. The following provides an example from a (fictional) annotated middle-author paper.

Forte, C., **Smith, J.**,* & Klein, A. (2011). Adrenal gland dysfunction in patients with vascular dementia. *International Journal of Dementia Research*, 43(7), 29–38.

*Conducted patient interviews and statistical analysis of data and drafted sections of the manuscript.

In some situations, a brief "blanket" description of authorship practices may obviate the need to annotate individual bibliographic citations. For example, consider a physician whose role is the same across multiple collaborative works and who participates extensively in the organization and performance of multicenter clinical trials coordinated by a national group. For this academic faculty member, relevant bibliographic entries might reference a single footnote briefly describing the recurrent individual role in trial design, implementation, analysis, and authorship.

The Bio Sketch

Many research grant and award applications require a bio sketch, much like a shortened version of the CV that summarizes your training and experiences. With more experienced applicants who have extensive publications, the bio sketch can be used to highlight specific nuances of the academic's expertise as relevant to a particular grant application. The National Institutes of Health provides an overview of the bio sketch on its Web site (see Further Reading at the end of this chapter). A newer addition to the bio sketch in the last few years is the personal statement.

The Personal Statement

Almost every application process requires a personal or autobiographical statement, whether as a separate document or in the form of a cover letter. The personal statement in an NIH bio sketch is meant to summarize the academic physician's experience and expertise in a relevant field and succinctly convey his or her particular value to an intended proposal [4]. Generally speaking, a personal statement serves to complement and supplement the CV with a description of the academic physician's qualifications and strengths in narrative form. Like a CV, the personal statement is written for a specific purpose or position, and it aims to convey to the reader how and why the academic physician is qualified for the position to which he or she is applying. The academic physician may want to emphasize the reason for his or her interest in a particular specialty at a particular program or institute.

The personal statement should highlight items in the CV that make the academic faculty member well prepared for a particular position. It is the physician's opportunity to expand upon activities listed in the CV but deserving of greater description so that the reader can appreciate the breadth and depth of one's involvement in the proposed study. The academic physician may also choose to relate significant personal experiences, but only if they are relevant to the application. Lastly, the personal statement is the appropriate place to specify one's professional goals. It offers the opportunity to outline clear, realistic, and carefully considered goals that will leave the reader with a strong impression of one's maturity, self-awareness, and character.

The importance of good writing skills for the personal statement cannot be overemphasized. The quality of the writing in the personal statement is at least as important as its content. Be sure to write in complete sentences and avoid abbreviations, repetitive sentence structure, and jargon. Use a dictionary, thesaurus, and spell-check program. Remember, in the early part of one's academic progress, the personal statement is the closest thing the reviewers have to knowing the academic faculty member personally.

Words to the Wise
- Remember that an application form is limited to the few things that a particular institution wants to know about everybody, whereas the CV allows the opportunity to present information that is unique. Add all key accomplishments and activities in the initial draft. In subsequent drafts, remove information that may not be pertinent.
- Resist the temptation to append explanatory sentences or language, which will distract the reader from the basic information being presented. The language of a CV should be abbreviated and succinct. Express yourself in the personal or biographical statement.
- Be honest! If accomplishments are lacking in a particular category, leave out the category rather than try to create accomplishments to fill in the space. Be specific about the level of participation in a project or an activity, but avoid being misleading.
- Remember that first impressions leave lasting memories. Typographical and grammatical errors, inconsistent formatting, and other presentation flaws reflect poorly on the academic faculty member. Be sure to closely review the final CV draft, and seek editorial scrutiny where possible. Ask colleagues and/or mentors to review the CV and provide additions and revisions.

Ask Your Mentor or Colleagues
- Can you look over my CV and give me feedback on its content and format?
- What strengths and weakness do you feel are reflected in my CV?
- Do you think I am on track for success? If not, what would you recommend that I do?
- Are there any institutional or other professional resources that you suggest I utilize to help me reach my academic goals?

Appendix: Sample CV

Janet Doe, **M.D.**
101 Main Street
San Francisco, CA
Phone: 555-555-5555
Cell: 555-666-6666
E-mail: email@email.com

PROFESSIONAL EXPERIENCE

Attending Physician
1990 to present
San Francisco General Hospital
San Francisco, CA
Assistant Professor
1990–1998
Department of Psychiatry
University of California, San Francisco
Associate Professor
1998 to present
Department of Psychiatry
University of California, San Francisco

EDUCATION

B.S. in Biology, 1982
University of California, Berkeley
M.D., 1986
Stanford University School of Medicine

Residency in Psychiatry, 1986–1990
San Francisco General Hospital
Fellowship in Child and Adolescent Psychiatry, 1991–1992
San Francisco General Hospital

CREDENTIALS

American Board of Psychiatry and Neurology
Board-Certified in Psychiatry, 1990
Board-Certified in Child and Adolescent Psychiatry, 1993
California Medical License #ABC123, 1986

BIBLIOGRAPHY

Peer-Reviewed Publications

Miller S, **Doe** J, Johnson D. (2007). Psychiatric medication efficacy in toddlers. *Journal of Family Practice, 23*, 1–14.

Doe J, Smith A. (2008). A community study to preventing drug abuse in children. *Journal of Drug Abuse Research, 17*, 22–30.

Presentations

"Conduct Disorder and Drugs of Abuse"
Annual Meeting of the American Psychiatric Association
May, 2006
"Current Treatment Models for Adolescent Drug Abuse"
East Bay Community Foundation
February, 2008

TEACHING AND MENTORING

Instructor, *Introduction to Clinical Interviewing* (Medical Students)
Fall semester of 2005, 2006, 2007
Department of Psychiatry
University of California, San Francisco
Mentor, McCarthy Medical Scholars Program
2005 to present
University of California, San Francisco
Course Director, *Pediatric Psychopharmacology* (Psychiatry Residents)
2007 to present
Department of Psychiatry
University of California, San Francisco

PROFESSIONAL MEMBERSHIPS AND SERVICE

Member

2000 to present, American Medical Association
2005 to present, US Psychiatric Association
2007 to present, US Association of Women in Psychiatry

Service
2005 to present, Manuscript Reviewer, *Journal of Alcohol Research*
2009–2011, Grant Reviewer, Foundation for Drug Abuse Research

References

1. Boss JM, Eckert SH. Academic scientists at work. 2nd ed. San Francisco, CA: Springer; 2006.
2. Simpson D, Hafler J, Brown D, Wilkerson L. Documentation systems for educators seeking academic promotion in U.S. medical schools. Acad Med. 2004;79(8):783–90.
3. Epstein D, Kenway J, Boden R. Academic's support kit—Writing for publication. London, UK: Sage; 2005.
4. Gerin W, Kapelewski CH. Writing the NIH grant proposal—A step-by-step guide. 2nd ed. London, UK: Sage; 2010.

Further Reading

National Institutes of Health Office of Intramural Training & Education: https://www.training.nih.gov/careers/careercenter
National Institutes of Health bio sketch samples: http://grants.nih.gov/grants/funding/phs398/phs398.html
Purdue Online Writing Lab: http://owl.english.purdue.edu/owl/resource/642/01/

How to Understand Promotion Criteria for "Clinician Educator" and "Teaching" Tracks

17

Michelle Goldsmith

My greatest moments as a teacher are when one of my mentees has internalized my belief in them so they can face a patient with the courage of their convictions and say what needs to be said without fear that they will make a fool of themselves. [1]

Glen O. Gabbard

Clinical educators transmit a body of clinical skills and core values from one generation to the next. Clinical educators can transform the medical school experience into an apprenticeships by providing face-to-face, immediate, one-on-one teaching—at the bedside, in the clinic, and in countless hours of formal and informal teaching. There are few professions that still offer this rich and varied learning environment. Moreover, clinician educators have a unique opportunity to integrate their knowledge, skills, and values into institutional curricula, thereby benefitting future generations.

M. Goldsmith, M.D., M.A. (✉)
Division of Child and Adolescent Psychiatry, Department of Psychiatry and Behavioral Health Sciences, Lucile Packard Children's Hospital/ Stanford Hospital and Clinics, 401 Quarry Road, Stanford, CA, USA
e-mail: michelle.goldsmith@stanford.edu

© Springer International Publishing Switzerland 2016
L.W. Roberts (ed.), *The Clinician Educator Guidebook*,
DOI 10.1007/978-3-319-27980-0_17

The value of clinical educators to their institutions is more difficult to quantify compared to the number grants and publications produced by their research-focused colleagues. Therefore, clinical educators often worry about their chances for promotion, their ability to thrive in the academic medical environment, and their capacity to deliver high-quality teaching during demanding times [2, 3]. Since clinical and educational programs are central components of academic medical institutions, retaining motivated, skilled, and dedicated clinical educators is a high priority for most institutions. For clinical educators, surviving and thriving in the academic environment requires more than being a skilled clinician and teacher. It is imperative to know how to navigate the academic environment— understanding promotion criteria is a *sine qua non* for professional success and fulfillment. To that end, this chapter provides a framework for understanding the clinical educator promotion criteria and offers suggestions on how to prepare for promotion.

The Clinical Educator: Definition and Expectations

Prior to the mid-1980s, the "triple threat" faculty member who excelled in research, teaching, and clinical care was one model for success. Due to increased competition for funding, challenges in measuring teaching efficacy, and the pressures of meeting clinical productivity requirements, faculty gravitated towards distinct roles of clinician–educators or clinician–researcher [5, 6]. Similarly, medical institutions, in response to trends in academia [7] and to generate funds to support medical education [4], distinguished between teaching and research positions by developing specific career paths for clinician educators. From 1986 to 2005, the number of academic medical institutions with clinical educator promotion and tenure tracks nearly doubled from 61 to 100 [4, 8].

Currently, the faculty handbooks of most academic medical centers include definitions for the clinician educator also known as academic educator, teaching scholar, or clinician-teacher. The definition of clinical educator varies widely, so as mentioned in previous chapters, you should consult your institution's faculty handbook to understand how clinician educators are defined within your institution. The information provided in this chapter describes normative definitions and is not meant to reflect all possible definitions. It is important to note that the documented description may not entirely reflect the dynamic clinician educator role with all of its nuances. To determine what your institution expects is best accomplished by speaking with those within your institution who have successfully attained promotion.

On the surface, the clinical educator is someone who is primarily engaged in clinical care and teaching that advances the field of clinical medicine with evidence of excellence in their duties. For some institutions, clinical educators also engage in scholarly activities and serve in administrative and leadership roles, for others, it is a requirement for advancement. Therefore, clinical educators distinguish themselves in four domains—clinical care, teaching, administration/leadership, and scholarship. These performance areas are the benchmarks commonly used to demonstrate high achievement and form the basis for promotion (see Table 17.1 for instruments used to assess performance areas).

Specific Expectations by Performance Area

Clinical Care

The academic medical community regards successful clinical educators as beyond competent and as models of excellence in clinical care. The guiding principle for who is considered to be an exemplary clinical educator is often "The doctor to whom you would refer your family member." Clinical educators differ in their clinical focus (generalist vs. specialist), ratio of responsibilities (clinical and teaching vs. clinical and administration), and the modalities by which they demonstrate their skills (teaching trainees clinical skills vs. patient education). Above all else, clinical educators demonstrate superb clinical care through accepted clinical proficiencies such as maintaining an up-to-date knowledge base of evidence-based practice and current standards of care, applying sound diagnostic and therapeutic reasoning and judgment, seeking consultation from other care providers and colleagues, meeting productivity requirements, and demonstrating reliability in meeting clinical commitments.

Table 17.1 Areas of performance and methods of documentation for clinical educators

Clinical care	Curriculum vitae (CV)
	Letters of reference from colleagues or mentees
	Peer evaluations
	Trainee evaluations
	Record of clinical productivity
	Physician referrals and written recommendations
	Patient feedback
	Clinical competency evaluations
	Development of a program to improve the quality of clinical care, meet an institutional need, or improve clinical outcome with data
Teaching	CV
	Letters of reference from colleagues or mentees
	Peer evaluations
	Trainee evaluations
	Teaching awards
	Timely supervisee feedback
	Documentation of learner achievement: residency match, job, scholarship
	Educator's portfolio
	Educational philosophy statement
	Short- and long-term goals as an educator
	Lists of supervisees, medical students taught and time spent
	Educational contributions by category:
	1. Teaching
	2. Learner assessment
	3. Curriculum development
	4. Mentoring and advising
	5. Educational leadership and administration
Administration/ leadership	CV
	Letters of reference from colleagues or mentees
	Peer evaluation
	Committee membership, leadership roles, documentation of completed work
	Documentation of positive change due to programs of benefit to clinical care, teaching, or institutional goals e.g. quality improvement measures

(continued)

Table 17.1 (continued)

Scholarship	CV
	List of peer reviewed publications
	Letters of reference from colleagues, mentees, or research mentors
	Peer reviewed publications cited by others
	Documented use of novel teaching or research tools used by other educators
	Grants or other sources of funding, e.g. your institution or professional society
	Professional society membership, committee membership, leadership role in either and documentation of accomplishments
	Accepted abstracts/presentations/workshops at other institutions, community health care organizations, professional societies
	Peer reviewer for journal/journal editor

Teaching

Well trained and experienced clinical educators teach with carefully developed lectures, newly designed curricula, and innovative modalities and materials. Frequently having obtained additional training in effective teaching, these doctors (from *docere*, Latin "to teach") apply criteria from educational scholarship to their teaching. The key components of teaching include clear goals, adequate preparation, appropriate methods, significant results, and effective reflection [7].

Proof of excellence in formal didactics and "bedside" teaching should be amassed through teaching evaluations from a variety of learners (e.g., visiting and native medical students; residents and fellows from within and external to your department; colleagues who are care providers, learners, or approached to serve as neutral observers; audiences at grand rounds, patient education seminars, professional societies; and other allied professionals). Strong teaching evaluations serve as a metric for assessing teaching competence, which is then used to evaluate readiness for promotion.

Administrative and Leadership Roles

Often accomplished clinical educators step into administrative and leadership roles in clinical care, education, and scholarship within their institution. Faculty often seek or are identified by department leadership to seek responsibilities that will allow them to expand their work and influence. The types of responsibilities vary and include roles such as membership on a hospital committee for quality improvement in emergency room services, interviewer for residency and fellowship applicants, and Director for medical education. Pursuing leadership positions in service to your institution, a professional society, or the community is a creative opportunity to develop your professional interests and goals. At the same time, these efforts support your promotion application, help others, and improve the quality of clinical academic medicine through dissemination of knowledge and services. The nature of administrative and leadership positions can differ (i.e., not all administrative tasks are characterized by leadership and vice versa). Regardless of how you choose to distinguish yourself, your application should provide evidence that your efforts have met a departmental or institutional need and add value.

Scholarship

Successful clinical educators develop a body of scholarly work to share with others via peer-reviewed journals, presenting seminars or lectures, conducting workshops at professional meetings, or public speaking in community settings. In the academic medical literature, the term scholarship, as it applies to the work of clinical educators, has undergone a shift in focus. Several organizations and authors have suggested that the parameters regarding content be widened beyond research with original data to capture scholarly efforts addressing educational methods of teaching, applications to clinical care, and cross disciplinary efforts [7, 9].

A newer definition of scholarship also refers to work which is readily available to the public, subject to peer review and critique according to accepted standards, and is reproduced as well as foundational to other scholars [10]. For example, a publication highlighting a new curriculum for teaching culturally competent clinical skills to medical students that was piloted at one institution, and then used at multiple academic centers with proven results in improving clinical care (pre- and post-measures) would meet the criteria at most institutions for high quality scholarship produced by a clinical educator.

In summary, developing a rich blend of skills in clinical care, teaching, administration/leadership, and scholarship requires clearly defined professional goals, and a systematic plan for academic achievement rooted in an understanding of the criteria for appointment, reappointment, and promotion. The clinical educator track at your institution may contain ranks requiring increasing demonstration of expertise in clinical care and teaching paired with evidence of scholarship and leadership. The rungs of this ranking ladder may be instructor, assistant clinical professor, associate clinical professor, and clinical professor. These titles differ across institutions and whether the position confers tenure (a secured position if promotion is achieved) varies at each institution. Importantly, the tenured clinical educator track is atypical and this detail should be clarified at the time of appointment. Most positions have fixed terms and can be renewed without limit, if an individual is meeting the job requirements. Whichever type of position (tenured or non-tenured track), the initial appointment is not a life-time guarantee, therefor reappointment and promotion require that you continue to develop your skills and demonstrate excellence.

Promotion Criteria

Self-Reflection

Preparation for promotion begins before your first day on the job. Planning your career path based on your interests and goals, and the needs of the institution, requires self-knowledge, strong mentorship, and openness to seeking information, and advice from others. At the outset, each candidate should carefully reflect on their accomplishments, and also any deficits (see Table 17.2 for a list of questions to consider). First, it is important to begin with self inquiry about professional goals which all

Table 17.2 Questions to ask oneself prior to eligibility for promotion by area of performance

Professional goals	*Career path*
	What motivates me?
	What are my strengths and limitations? Do I want to change them and how?
	What would I like to be doing in 5 years on a daily basis? How am I making this happen?
	Curriculum vitae (CV)
	How is my CV: gaps, format, meeting institutional standards, clarity? Does my CV reflect what I really do?
	Do I update my CV regularly as I do things or just when I need to circulate my CV?
	Do I have different versions of my CV for different purposes: promotion, bio sketch, recruitment?
	Networking
	How am I perceived by others in the workplace?
	Who are my stakeholders and supporters? How do they help or hurt me?
	What professional organizations can I join and how can I contribute to them to develop a regional and national reputation regarding clinical care, teaching, and/or scholarship?
	How can I cultivate relationships extra-departmentally to build my local reputation?
	Mentorship
	Who are my mentors?
	How is the fit?
	What are my goals in working with these mentors?
	Do my mentors represent my different areas of interest?
Clinical care	What is my focus and area of concentration?
	Do I have all of my peer and/or patient evaluations? Do they measure my contribution and if not what else can I do?
	In what way have I improved clinical care at my institution?
	What is my philosophy regarding patient care?

(continued)

Table 17.2 (continued)

Teaching	What is my focus and area of concentration?
	What is my philosophy on teaching?
	Do I have all of my teaching evaluations from peers and/or trainees? Do they measure my contribution and if not what else can I do?
	Have I regularly pursued teaching/mentoring of students and documented those activities and student outcomes?
	What educational programs can I design that will improve current teaching or learning for peers or trainees?
	Have I taken advantage of opportunities to advance my teaching skills?
Scholarship	What is my focus and area of concentration?
	To what extent am I recognized as an expert or highly excelled?
	How have I documented my leadership and eligibility for awards with regard to scholarship?
	What opportunities exist to talk and teach externally (e.g., CME, Grand Rounds), and to write in peer-reviewed national contexts?
	What peer reviewed projects can I collaborate on or initiate? Could any include original data?
	Is my work reproducible and helpful to other educators?
	Do I want to apply for funding to support scholarship which may free up some of my time?
	Have I taken advantage of opportunities to advance my research skills?
Leadership/ administration	What is my focus and area of concentration?
	Do my goals and contribution meet an institutional need?
	Have I taken advantage of opportunities to be in a leadership role, contribute to the institution, and to heighten my visibility?
	How is my leadership and contribution recognized and documented?
	How can I improve or broaden my administrative and leadership skills?

faculty should address regardless of their rank, aspirations, or track. By answering these questions in writing (your answers may change over time), you will create direction for your career and take control of your path rather than finding yourself in an undesirable circumstance.

Self-reflection can be challenging and may require some informal or professional coaching. As with any other area of your life, your career deserves attention and resources. Although time and money spent on your professional development is your responsibility, most academic medical centers set aside resources to support you. Do not give away "free" money earmarked to cultivate your professional skills. Asking your department to invest in you (e.g., sponsoring professional society membership, travel funds to lecture, sponsorship for conferences to improve your teaching, or research skills) is a reasonable request.

Self-reflection for some individuals comes through phoning a friend. Identify "buddies" (i.e., trusted individuals offering candid feedback and insight from their own experience) who will be your sounding board and provide you with guidance. Having at least one buddy at your home institution, and another at a comparable academic medical center, ensures multiple perspectives with and without the bias of your workplace. Other aspiring faculty members contact the office of career development at their institution, meet with senior faculty, and consult with mentors for career counseling. Support from others during the promotion process starts with gathering advice and counsel; be thoughtful and careful about what you share and with whom you share it.

Process

After the decision has been made to proceed with the promotion process, you will typically have contact with the administrator in your department who handles promotion requests. Some institutions require that you request promotion in writing directed to your division chair or supervisor, while other institutions initiate the promotion process on your behalf. A summary memo, or letter of recommendation, is generated by your department for the departmental clinical educator appointment and promotion (A&P)

committee to review along with your current CV. The A&P committee will make a decision as to whether or not they recommend promotion. This decision is given to the department chair for review. If your promotion is recommended and approved by the department chair, your file is forwarded to the school of medicine's clinical educator A&P committee to evaluate your entire promotion "package."

The "Package"

In the "package" or promotion application, the A&P committee will find your updated CV, a summary of your job responsibilities, internal and external letters of reference, and your teaching and clinical evaluations. In some cases, a package will also contain a candidate statement, an educator portfolio, and evaluation forms from colleagues attesting to clinical excellence in core competencies.

A candidate statement is not always a requirement. It may be requested for those pursuing more senior rank and optional for more junior faculty. A candidate statement is approximately two pages, written in the first person, and discusses your contributions and achievements broken down by area of performance. It may also include background on prior accomplishments, highlights of current work, and a summary of goals for future endeavors. A strong candidate statement provides a context for the entire promotion packet and coupled with a teacher's portfolio provides examples of your educational contribution.

When required, teaching portfolios typically include a statement of the clinical educator's teaching philosophy, short- and long-term goals, references for supervisees and mentees, and samples of teaching, learner feedback and assessment, curricula developed, and teaching material such as syllabi, and course descriptions or novel materials. Examples of candidate statements and portfolios can be found on-line (see Further Reading at the end of this chapter).

In conclusion, consider your application an opportunity to pitch yourself to the A&P committee. Design a thoughtfully prepared "story" (candidate statement) describing your unique blend of

Table 17.3 Components of the promotion application or "package"

Common items

1. Letter of recommendation from division chief or supervisor
2. Job description/responsibilities
3. Updated and verified curriculum vitae
4. Internal and external letters of reference
5. Teaching evaluations
6. Clinical evaluations

Possible items

1. Candidate statement
2. Educator's teaching portfolio
3. Evaluation of institutional core competencies completed by colleagues, allied health professionals, referring physician, trainees

skills and accomplishments, and support it with evidence from your portfolio, letters of reference, and evaluations all of which are a testament to your accomplishments (Table 17.3).

> **Key Concepts**
> - Know the specific criteria and procedures for promotion at your institution.
> - If your contribution is not documented, it will not count significantly in the promotion process.
> - Continuously develop your CV, promotion package, and essential skills for demonstrating excellence in clinical care and teaching.
> - Regularly consult with other peers, mentors, and colleagues to assess your professional development.
> - Be aware of the departmental and institutional politics that may influence your candidacy for promotion.

Controversies and Opportunities

Most clinical educators care for patients approximately 80 % of the time though this can vary widely. This distribution creates a challenge whereby clinical educators feel that they do not have enough time to engage in high quality teaching while maintaining excellent clinical care. One possible strategy for those that feel time pressed is to incorporate teaching as much as possible into patient care by having trainees present when seeing patients. Whether the bedside, operating room, or outpatient clinics, these settings afford ample opportunity to teach about evidence-based care to the next generation of doctors. If this sort of teaching is not available to you and you are providing formal didactics on a regular basis then you may want to carefully consider requesting that your job description be altered and provide support for your request.

Time demands on clinical educators can be significant. The high volume of patients coupled with the complex task of consistently providing high quality teaching, and remaining current with advances in medicine can be overwhelming. Moreover, lack of protected time to devote to scholarly work can lead to faculty becoming dissatisfied with their careers. As the clinical educator track evolves, institutions and leaders in medical education are acknowledging the need for different types of clinical educators and ways of defining and achieving success [9, 11, 12]. In addition to institutional support for change, clinical educators will need to be creative by strategizing and working "smarter not harder" to achieve their academic goals. For example, assigning brief presentations to trainees on advancements in clinical care will provide you with new information and an opportunity to teach trainees how to search the literature, present material, and perhaps develop into a writing project. In conclusion, having a clear understanding of the promotion criteria for the clinical educator role will support your efforts to advance your career in academic medicine. Each individual should gravitate towards those aspects of their job which are the most gratifying but avoid neglecting less desirable activities. To the best of your ability design your job to allow yourself opportunities in the areas which you find most meaningful and serve the mission of your institution. Then you will find joy in your work and be recognized and rewarded both personally and professionally.

Words to the Wise
- Consult with clinical educators who have sought promotion from your department, in other departments at your institution, and at other institutions.
- Consult with your mentors about each aspect of your promotion packet, your candidate statement, selecting your letters of reference, and the strengths and vulnerabilities of your promotion application.
- Learn who is on the promotion committee in your department and for the institution. Research their backgrounds and meet with individuals to discuss the promotion process.
- Determine how faculty in your track are valued and recognized at your institution. In addition, learn how you can contribute to the institution's mission of clinical care and teaching.
- To create a "fit" between you and your employer, you must understand the unwritten rules of promotion which requires honest self-reflection, assertiveness, savvy, and professional behavior in all aspects of your work.
- Avail yourself of further developmental opportunities to cultivate your clinical, teaching, scholarly, and leadership skills by investing time to get training and experience in adult education.
- Take responsibility for the distribution and collection of evaluations every time you teach.

Ask Your Mentor or Colleagues
- What is my timeline for promotion?
- Where do I stand in relation to my peers within the department, institution, and at other comparable academic centers?
- How would I "package" myself at this point in time? What will my "narrative" be?
- How do clinical educators develop a regional and national reputation at this institution?

Further Reading

Electronic Handbooks

For clinical educators:
  http://www.bcm.edu/pediatrics/?pmid=16210
  http://download.book5.org/m/medical-school-based-career-and-leadership-development-programs-w1333.html
  For trainees:
  http://familymed.uthscsa.edu/ACE/pdf_chapters/Guidebook_Chp12.pdf
  Articles on clinical care, teaching and research for clinical educators

- Kroenke K. Conducting research as a busy clinician-teacher or trainee: starting blocks, hurdles, and finish lines. J Gen Intern Med. 1996;11:360–65.
- Ende J. What if Osler were one of us? Inpatient teaching today. J Gen Intern Med. 1997;12 Suppl 2:S41–S8.
- McGee SR, Irby DM. Teaching in the outpatient clinic. Practical tips. J Gen Intern Med. 1997;12 Suppl 2:S34–S40.
- Zerzan JT, Hess R, Schur E, Phillips RS, Rigotti N. Making the most of mentors: a guide for mentees. Acad Med. 2009;84 Suppl 1:140–4.
- Detsky AS, Baerlocher MO. Academic mentoring—how to give it and how to get it. JAMA. 2007;297:2134–36.

University Websites

UMDNJ:
  http://cte.umdnj.edu/clinical_education/index.cfm

Harvard:
  http://www.bidmc.org/MedicalEducation/AcademicCareersandFacultyDevelopment.aspx

Southern Illinois University:
  http://www.siumed.edu/dme/academy/medical_education.html

Other Website Resources

https://www.mededportal.org/

Examples of the educator's portfolio:
https://www.aamc.org/members/gfa/faculty_vitae/148574/educator_portfolio.html

http://www.ambpeds.org/education/educator_portfolio_template.cfm

https://www.aamc.org/members/gfa/faculty_vitae/150038/cv_cv_portfolio.html

References

1. Gabbard G. Why I, teach. Acad Psychiatry. 2011;35(5):277–82.
2. Kumar K, Roberts C, Thistlethwaite J. Entering and navigating academic medicine: academic clinician-educators' experiences. Med Educ. 2011;45(5):497–503.
3. Dahlstrom J, Dorai-Raj A, McGill D, Owen C, Tymms K, Watson DA. What motivates senior clinicians to teach medical students? BMC Med Educ. 2005;5(1):27.
4. Kelley WN, Stross JK. Faculty tracks and academic success. Ann Intern Med. 1992;116(8):654–9.
5. Glassick CE. Boyer's expanded definitions of scholarship, the standards for assessing scholarship, and the elusiveness of the scholarship of teaching. Acad Med. 2000;75(9):877–80.
6. Alexander H. Report on faculty tracks with research expectations. Washington, DC: Association of American Medical Colleges; 2005.
7. Lubitz RM. Guidelines for promotion of clinician-educators. The society of general internal medicine education committee. J Gen Intern Med. 1997;12 Suppl 2:S71–S8.
8. Hutchings P, Shulman LS. The scholarship of teaching: new elaborations, new developments. Change. 1999;31(5):10–5.
9. Durso SC, Christmas C, Kravet SJ, Parsons G, Wright SM. Implications of academic medicine's failure to recognize clinical excellence. Clin Med Res. 2009;7(4):127–33.
10. Carey RM, Wheby MS, Reynolds RE. Evaluating faculty clinical excellence in the academic health sciences center. Acad Med. 1993;68(11):813–7.
11. Collins J. The needs of an educator. J Am Coll Radiol. 2005; 2(11):914–8.
12. Richards BF, Moran BJ, Friedland JA, Kirkland RT, Searle NS, Coburn M. A criterion-based, peer review process for assessing the scholarship of educational leadership. Acad Med. 2002;77(10):S7–9.

How to Create Your Package for Promotion

18

Judith P. Cain and David K. Stevenson

From the perspective of the candidate, the pathways leading to the promotion review—as well as the review itself—are often seen as mysterious and confusing. This observation was confirmed in a 2008 study conducted by the Collaborative on Academic Careers in Higher Education (COACHE) [1] in which pre-tenure faculty at medical schools and health professions gave low ratings to the level of clarity surrounding tenure processes, criteria, standards, and the body of evidence needed for promotion.

Some of this mystery and confusion is complicated by the subjective, evaluative aspect of promotion standards. In that respect, there are no easy answers to such questions as the following: How many peer-reviewed articles do I need? When, what, and where should I publish? What types of grants and how much funding should I have? How many students should I be teaching and mentoring? What ratings do I have to have on my teaching and clinical evaluations? Also, academic careers tend to be individualized in terms of breadth, depth, and focus, resulting in multiple pathways

J.P. Cain (✉)
Department of Medicine, Stanford University, 1265 Welch Road, Stanford, CA, USA
e-mail: jpcain@stanford.edu

© Springer International Publishing Switzerland 2016
L.W. Roberts (ed.), *The Clinician Educator Guidebook*,
DOI 10.1007/978-3-319-27980-0_18

to success. Thus, it is difficult, if not impossible, to draw a specific road map that can be universally applied to all faculty that will predict or guarantee a successful promotion outcome.

The application of promotion criteria is usually centered on expectations for excellence in a particular faculty line. For example, in the tenure line, a greater proportional weight may be given to scholarship than in a more clinically-oriented line where there may be a balance between clinical care, teaching, and scholarly activities; in some lines, senior-authored, peer-reviewed publications are the *coin of the realm*, while in others there may be more flexibility in considering collaborative work, case reports, invited chapters, textbooks, or conference proceedings. Chapters 17 and 18 provide guidance in understanding criteria for *traditional*, *research*, *clinical educator*, and *teaching* tracks. In addition to evaluating achievements against the criteria for a specific line, those reviewing the promotion package will be assessing the relative placement within a field or subfield nationally; Chap. 20 will be helpful in mapping out a plan to build a national reputation.

Given that there is no single prescribed, quantifiable path to promotion, perceptions regarding criteria and standards can be influenced by a variety of experiences, both personal and professional. As a result, different things may be said by different people about what is needed to advance in rank. While it will be important to gather perspectives from a variety of individuals in the years leading up to the promotion review, under most circumstances—and since the review will be initiated at the departmental level—the department chair is in the best position to provide guidance and counsel, to confirm current standards, and to interpret how the criteria will be applied in considering a particular case for promotion.

Institutional Responsibility

Institutions share the common goal of creating a culture and building an environment in which their faculty can develop, flourish, and succeed. In response to the COACHE study, and as part of a continuing commitment to enhance professional development opportunities for early-career faculty, many institutions have made it a priority to promote accessibility, clarity, and transparency in promotion reviews. Toward that end, efforts have included making policy documents (such as faculty handbooks) widely and easily available; offering university-, school-, or department-sponsored workshops on promotion criteria and processes; developing flexible workplace arrangements that may include extension of the promotion clock; initiating annual pre-promotion discussions between the department chair (or designate) and the early-career faculty member in order to regularly assess the candidate's progress toward promotion; providing training sessions for departmental, school, and university review committees; and actively protecting and preserving the integrity of the evaluation process by carefully following standardized procedures.

Of course, institutional responsibility is also carried out on a more direct and personal level. Through its decision to hire a new faculty member, the department has expressed its confidence not only in the individual's past and present achievements but also in his or her promise for the future. Because of this investment in the faculty member's success, the department chair, senior colleagues, and mentors will be partners in his or her professional development, providing support and honest assessment of career development and progress as the person moves through the early years of appointment.

Faculty Responsibility

While institutions have certain obligations, it is important for faculty to understand that they must be active in preparing for promotion and take responsibility for their career trajectory. As the primary stakeholder in the process, faculty should actively seek out information that will assist in the promotion process. The investment of time and effort in learning as much as possible about what is expected can pay dividends later. The confidence that comes with understanding the promotion process will enable faculty to put forth a promotion package that makes a compelling case for advancement.

Building a Strong Foundation of Knowledge

It is always a good idea to establish a baseline of information early. Candidates should reread their offer letter for details about faculty line, responsibilities, appointment term, and criteria for reappointment or promotion. They should study their institution's faculty handbook (usually readily available online), which will be an invaluable resource in providing information about the fundamentals of criteria, policies, and procedures. School or departmental websites may also provide useful information, especially with respect to any supplemental practices at those levels. A variety of other information may also be posted on these websites, such as the components of the promotion package (including the candidate's contributions), sample letters used in soliciting evaluations from referees and trainees, sample teaching and clinical evaluation forms, and timelines. If anything is unclear, especially regarding promotion criteria, the candidate should seek out answers from departmental leadership sooner rather than later.

Although the actual promotion review may be years in the future, it is important that the candidate systematically records and tracks relevant achievements as they occur. Faculty at many institutions have access to vendor or in-house web databases for the creation of e-portfolios. This is an efficient and productive way to store and update the curriculum vitae, annual activity reports, and other information on scholarly, teaching, and clinical activities that will be needed for the midterm and promotion reviews. Understanding the scope of and required formats for these materials will allow the candidate to collect and organize information cumulatively rather than at the last minute.

As mentioned previously, many institutions offer orientations or regular workshops for faculty focusing on such topics as promotion criteria, timing, and dossier preparation. Candidates for promotion should make every effort to participate in such sessions; if they are unable to attend, they should ask for copies of the slides or handouts from the meeting and follow up with questions, if necessary. They should also be alert to other workshops that may be held on such topics as time management, work–life balance, negotiating skills, and networking within and beyond the boundaries of their institution, all of which are aimed at enhancing professional development and success as a member of the academic community.

Annual meetings with the department chair or designate will provide a regular opportunity to discuss and measure progress against criteria for promotion. If such annual meetings are not common practice in their department, faculty members should initiate them. This is particularly important in the early years of the appointment since such sessions will provide ample time to address any issues and, if necessary, make course corrections well in advance of the promotion review. Mentors can also provide guidance and counsel and be good sounding boards as the candidate moves through the first, second, and third years of appointment.

The Midterm Review and Beyond

Typically, candidates will have a formal review of their performance near the midpoint of the appointment. For assistant professors who are on a 7-year appointment track, this review will be conducted in either the third or fourth year of appointment. At many institutions, the midterm evaluation is not as extensive as the promotion review but shares some of the same elements and thus can serve as a useful preview. Feedback from the review should be used to address any concerns and to build momentum that will carry the candidate through promotion review 3 or 4 years hence.

After the midterm review, efforts should be stepped up to gather perspectives that will be of value and benefit as the promotion review draws closer. Those who have invested in the candidate's success, including the department chair or division leader, senior colleagues, and mentors, will all be in a position to provide targeted, strategic counseling and feedback. Departmental or school administrative staff will be able to provide technical advice about the process. Colleagues within or outside the department who have recently been promoted may be willing to share their experiences. Senior faculty who have completed terms of service on school or university review committees may be able to provide insight into what distinguishes a superb promotion dossier from a weak one. It is important to note

Table 18.1 Sample pathway to the promotion review

Year 1	Re-read offer letter; study faculty handbook; review relevant websites, create an electronic portfolio to record and track achievements systematically
Year 2	Attend promotion workshops; meet frequently with mentor(s); meet with department chair annually to discuss progress toward promotion
Year 3	Understand policies regarding promotion clock extensions; prepare materials for midterm review
Year 4	Midterm review
Year 5	Incorporate and act on feedback from midterm review
Year 6	Continue regular meetings with mentor(s) and annual meetings with department chair; initiate conversations with those recently promoted; seek strategic advice from senior colleagues
Year 7	Begin preparation of promotion package; circulate CV and candidate's statement for feedback; submit promotion package

that under most circumstances, it is considered inappropriate to approach faculty currently serving in such a role and inquire about the disposition of a particular dossier (see Table 18.1).

Timing of the Promotion Review

In order to prepare for the promotion review, candidates need to be familiar with issues surrounding timing. The length of the appointment term—and therefore the timing of the promotion review—may depend on which faculty line the candidate is in. For example, in the School of Medicine at Stanford University, early-career faculty who are in the University Tenure Line (with a primary emphasis on research and teaching) typically have an initial appointment of 4 years followed by reappointment for 3 years; the tenure review is then initiated at the beginning of the seventh year in rank. Faculty in the Medical Center Line (where there is an expectation for excellence in the overall mix of clinical care, research, and teaching) are on a 10-year appointment clock, with an initial appointment of 4 years followed by a 6-year reappointment; the promotion review starts at the beginning of the tenth year.

At many institutions, there is often flexibility around extending the appointment end date for faculty who become new parents. Early on, faculty members should learn about this or any other circumstances that might result in favorable consideration of such an extension. On the other end of the spectrum, there may be flexibility regarding consideration for early promotion. Coming up early for promotion or extending the timing of the decision both require advance planning and close consultation with the department chair.

Typically, the promotion review will be launched up to 1 year in advance of the candidate's appointment end date. Timelines will vary institution by institution but are influenced by a common set of rate-limiting requirements, including the often lengthy process of soliciting and receiving letters from referees, students, and trainees; gathering, presenting, and evaluating evidence regarding scholarship, teaching, and clinical activities; and multiple levels of evaluation by departmental, school, and university review committees. All of this can and does take time. A sample timeline of the promotion process is included in the Appendix.

One of the topics at the midterm review should be the timing of the promotion review. Candidates will need to know not only the date when their department will formally launch the review but also the approximate deadline for submission of materials, which will allow them to plan accordingly. For example, if candidates are on a 7-year promotion clock, their review could be initiated as early as the *beginning* of the seventh year of appointment. Given the demands on their time, they should normally allow between 3 and 6 months to assemble the promotion package. They may need less, but it is better to provide the luxury of a *cushion*.

Candidates for promotion have the responsibility for designing and pursuing a schedule of research that results in publication in advance of the promotion review. Generally, by the time materials have been submitted, the candidate's dossier should predominantly reflect a record of actual accomplishment (which confirms status in the field) rather than work that has been submitted or accepted but not yet published (which may speak more to promise). Similarly, the faculty member's career should be managed so that teaching and clinical care records are robust and ready to be evaluated by the time that the promotion package is submitted.

Review committee members will expect expert referees to assess the candidate's impact and influence as a scholar through the lens of work that has been subjected to broad, formal scrutiny and cited by leaders in the field. Although unpublished work cannot be evaluated in the same way, it is important to document works in progress in the curriculum vitae and personal statement as this will be valuable in confirming momentum and upward trajectory.

Along with understanding the timing of the review, it is also important to be on time in submitting promotion materials. Candidate-driven delays can raise issues of professionalism at a highly inopportune time. If there are compelling reasons why a candidate is unable to meet any deadlines for submission of the dossier, the department chair should be informed immediately.

The Components of the Promotion Package

From evaluations by referees and students to departmental commentary and analysis of a candidate's contributions, there are many interconnected components of the promotion review. Its centerpiece, however, is the candidate's contribution, which provides an opportunity to both showcase accomplishments and to illuminate future plans. Sometimes called a *dossier* or *portfolio*, such contributions will typically include:

Curriculum Vitae

Chapter 16 of this book focuses on how to prepare the best possible curriculum vitae when joining a faculty. Building on that strong foundation, here are some things that candidates should consider when preparing a CV for the promotion review:

- Build the CV systematically and over time, using online tools to collect and track accomplishments and contributions.
- If the institution requires a standardized format, use it.
- Review sample CVs on departmental or school websites or ask recently promoted colleagues if they would be willing to share their CV.

- Distinguish between peer-reviewed and non-peer-reviewed publications and between invited presentations (even those declined) and *call for papers*. Those who will be reviewing the promotion package will be expecting this distinction, and not making it can create confusion or give the impression that the candidate is mischaracterizing his or her contributions.
- Authorship practices in many disciplines follow a traditional pattern in which the first author listed is the primary author and the last author listed is the senior author associated with the work. If practices differ in a discipline, this should be explained in a footnote or in the candidate's statement.
- Note which publications are in press and which have been submitted and to whom.
- For teaching contributions, use a broad definition that includes the classroom, laboratory or clinical setting, advising, mentoring, program building, and curricular innovation.
- In addition to clinical contributions that are reflected through scholarly and teaching activities, such things as medical consultancies, hospital appointments, and patents should be highlighted.
- There is a fine line between being comprehensive and padding the CV; candidates should learn the difference by concentrating on substantive contributions and, if uncertain, ask the department chair, mentor, or colleagues for advice.
- If responsibility for keeping the CV up to date has been delegated to administrative staff, candidates should remember that they are ultimately responsible for its content. The document should be read thoroughly and proofread by at least one other person.

With the increasing prevalence of *team science*, it can be challenging for committee reviewers to determine the nature of individual substantive contributions to multi-author works when reviewing a CV. Under such circumstances, candidates might want to consider briefly annotating selected bibliographic entries to highlight individual contributions to collaborative efforts.

A version of authorship requirements of the *Journal of the American Medical Association* [2], which includes the following categories, can be used as a model: (1) conception and design, acquisition of data and analysis and interpretation of data; (2) drafting of the manuscript and critical revision of the manuscript for important intellectual content; and (3) statistical analysis, obtaining funding, administrative, technical or material support, and supervision.

Candidates should anticipate that file reviewers will notice if there are unusual gaps in their CV and provide context for this in their candidate's statement. For example, a shift in research direction may have influenced productivity, the rate of publications flowing out of clinical trials may have been slowed due to lengthy periods of design and implementation, or sanctioned periods of protected time for research may have resulted in a reduced number of teaching opportunities. In providing this information, the tone should be explanatory and not defensive.

Candidate's Statement

Sometimes called the *personal* or *self* statement, this document serves as the candidate's voice in the promotion review and as a rich resource to those evaluating the case for promotion. In this narrative report, candidates will have an opportunity to discuss their accomplishments to date, the intersections of their scholarly, teaching, and clinical care contributions, and their plans for the future. Inclusion of a candidate's statement in the promotion package is sometimes optional but is almost always a good investment of time and effort. More often than not, institutions will have a required format, as well as page limitations. Knowing this well in advance will provide candidates with a framework in which to craft and effectively present their case for promotion.

There will be multiple audiences for the candidate's statement. Some readers, including departmental colleagues and external referees, will have expertise in and an understanding of the evolution of the candidate's discipline. Others, including members of school and university review committees, the dean, and the provost, may have homes in disciplines further removed from or entirely outside of academic medicine (such as physics, economics, or history). Because of this, candidates should take care to describe their accomplishments in lay terms that will be understandable and accessible to those outside their field.

With the caveat that the faculty member's department will be the primary source for information regarding the content and format of the candidate's statement, the following general guidelines may prove useful:

- While it is often appropriate to include contextual information regarding earlier contributions, it is usually important to concentrate on achievements made during the current term of appointment. For example, if the candidate is being reviewed at the beginning of the seventh year of appointment, accomplishments realized over the last 5 or 6 years may prove most relevant for purposes of evaluating satisfaction of criteria for promotion.
- In order to provide evaluators with a sense of career trajectory, it is important to include a discussion of near-term (e.g., works in progress), longer-range plans and goals for future work.
- Commentary should be included for each area on which the candidate will be evaluated, and the statement should be organized to align with the relative weight given to promotion criteria. For example, if the candidate will be evaluated primarily on clinical care activities (and, presumably, the highest proportion of time is dedicated to that area), the candidate's statement should begin with that and then, in descending order of weight and contribution, address other areas of contribution.
- The section on scholarly activities might include a general description of the overall investigative program, major contributions and accomplishments with particular emphasis on recent achievements, major publications and scientific discoveries and how they have impacted knowledge or further research in the field and/or patient care (including those that rank highly on citation indices), major grants and awards, and future goals, including ongoing research projects, publications planned for submission, and grant applications planned or in review.
- As mentioned previously, if authorship practices in the faculty member's discipline vary from the norm, this should be explained in the candidate's statement.
- The section on teaching might include commentary on clinical *bedside* teaching (e.g., medical students, residents, fellows, ancillary staff, and visiting or community physicians); didactic instruction, including informal lectures in the clinical setting,

formal classroom lectures, and continuing education; career mentoring and advising contributions; research mentoring and director supervision (undergraduate students, graduate students, postdoctoral fellows, medical students, residents, clinical fellows); prestigious positions obtained by former trainees; program or curriculum development; teaching awards; and future goals and plans.

– Commentary on clinical care activities could include discussion of the candidate's area of expertise and inpatient/outpatient/procedural contributions, percentages of time spent in clinic or the operating room, interaction with or consultation to other services, outreach contributions, development and/or implementation of new clinical trials or protocols and their real or potential impact, grand rounds, clinical care awards received, and future goals and plans.

– Some institutions protect early-career faculty from administrative commitments but, if relevant and applicable to promotion criteria, a description of service roles, responsibilities, and accomplishments should be included.

– In cases where promotion criteria include regional or national recognition, service positions (e.g., editorial or grant reviewer), major invited presentations or visiting professorships, conferences and symposia organized, and elected leadership positions and/or honors and awards from professional societies should be highlighted.

Sample Publications

Many institutions require or encourage submission of work, usually in the form of publications, as part of the promotion package. In some cases, such samples are shared locally, that is, with departmental faculty and/or departmental school and university evaluation committees. In other cases, a candidate's publications will also be sent to external referees. Since the number of publications to be submitted is usually limited, it is important that they be selected with thoughtfulness and care.

Normally, sample publications will be those that have appeared in print. Occasionally, however, there may be compelling reasons to include submitted or accepted publications that are unpublished at the time of the promotion review. Candidates are encouraged to seek guidance from the department chair, mentor, or senior colleagues in this matter.

Educator Portfolio

An *educator* or *teaching* portfolio is sometimes a required component of the promotion package. As with the curriculum vitae and candidate's statement, there may be a prescribed format, which should be followed closely. Chapter 19 of this book may be used as a guide in developing an educator portfolio.

Referees

Candidates for promotion are often asked to provide the names of leaders in the field who would be in a position to evaluate their work. The composition of the referee set varies by institution but may include a combination of mentors or collaborators of the candidate as well as those who are at *arm's length* and can provide independent perspectives. Colleagues within the candidate's institution may also be asked to provide a letter of evaluation.

For many reasons, including opportunities for advancement in their career, it is important for faculty members to be active and visible members of their discipline through participating in conferences and symposia, making presentations to national audiences, and serving on review panels and editorial boards. Likewise, it is crucial to establish, build, and sustain strong relationships with departmental colleagues and, given the evolving interdisciplinary nature of many fields, to make connections across other departments. Through such networking activities, the candidate will be well positioned to suggest the names of referees who are familiar with his or her work and will be able to provide a substantive and meaningful evaluation.

Post-submission of the Promotion Package

After materials have been submitted, departmental staff will contact the candidate if questions arise. If significant events—such as grants, publication acceptances, or awards—occur *after* the promotion package has been submitted, candidates should check with their department chair to see if there is a way for this information to become part of the record under review.

In the interest of transparency and clarity, the department chair should be able to provide the candidate with an approximate timeline for the final decision. Depending on an institution's policies, this could be either weeks or months, although the candidate may be informed at intervals as the review passes from one level to the next. Most institutions take extensive measures to protect the privacy of the candidate by preserving the confidentiality of the information it receives about him or her. At the same time, institutions expect that candidates will similarly respect the confidentiality of the process. Therefore, under normal circumstances, the candidate should not request or seek to discover confidential information from individuals within or outside the home institution who may be involved in the review process. The department chair will be in the best position to address any ambiguities or concerns the candidate might have in this regard.

Promotion Rates

Promotion rates are tracked in various ways. At Stanford University, data for faculty in the tenure line are organized by 5-year hire cohorts with outcomes across four categories (tenured, denied tenure, resigned, or other [including those who were to be reviewed at a future date]). For example, of the 107 tenure-line assistant professors hired into clinical and basic science departments from 1990 to 1999, 65 were granted tenure, 6 were denied tenure, 18 resigned, and 18 fell into other categories, which resulted, for that hire cohort, in a tenure rate of 60.7 %. However, when you isolate the 71 faculty who came up for tenure, the success rate rises to 92 %.

The Association of American Medical Colleges (AAMC) analyzes promotion rates for tenure track and non-tenure-track assistant and associate professors in a similar manner. The data are collected and analyzed through its Faculty Roster database, which is the only national database on the employment, training, and demographic background of US medical school faculty. Findings from this analysis were published in AAMC's Analysis in Brief, which included promotion rates for tenure and non-tenure-track assistant and associate professors, as well as the number of years to promotion (Table 18.2).

The relatively low promotion rates of 54.9 % for tenure track and 35.2 % for non-tenure-track assistant professors in the 1987–1993 hire cohort were likely influenced, as are the Stanford percentages, by the number of faculty who did not come up for promotion. For example, outcomes for a hire cohort of 120 assistant professors could include 70 faculty who were promoted, 20 faculty who were not promoted, and 30 faculty who, due to resignation or other factors, did not come up for promotion. In looking at the entire cohort, the promotion rate would be 58 %. However, the rate would rise to 78 % for actions in which a promotion decision was rendered. Generally, promotion rates are higher for those groups of faculty who successfully travel through their first and second terms as assistant professors and undergo the promotion review.

Data on national outcomes and trends are helpful to academic leaders in calibrating promotion rates at their own institutions. However, pathways to individual promotion reviews are as varied and unique as the candidates themselves. And outcomes are dependent upon many factors including, importantly, a strong partnership between the candidate and institution on which a successful case for promotion can be made.

Table 18.2 Promotion rates for tenure and non-tenure-track assistant and associate professors and number of years to promotion from AAMC's analysis in brief

Study group	First-time assistant professors						First-time associate professors					
	Average 10-year promotion rates			Average no. of years to promotion for promoted faculty			Average 10-year promotion rates			Average no. of years to promotion for promoted faculty		
	1967–1976 Cohorts	1977–1986 Cohorts	1987–1996 Cohorts	1967–1976 Cohorts	1977–1986 Cohorts	1987–1996 Cohorts	1967–1976 Cohorts	1977–1986 Cohorts	1987–1996 Cohorts	1967–1976 Cohorts	1977–1986 Cohorts	1987–1996 Cohorts
All faculty	43.5	40.4	32.8	5.2	5.8	6.2	41.7	42.6	38.6	5.7	5.9	6.1
Clinical departments												
M.D. or equivalent	44.7	39.4	31.2	5.1	5.8	6.3	44.1	43.1	37.8	5.6	5.9	6.2
Ph.D. or equivalent	37.9	37.6	30.8	5.6	5.8	6.3	28.9	35.3	33.0	6.0	6.2	6.2
M.D. and Ph.D. or equivalent	55.0	52.1	48.1	4.9	5.6	6.0	51.2	54.0	49.8	5.6	5.7	5.9
Basic sciences												
M.D. or equivalent	39.0	37.0	33.2	5.1	5.9	6.2	46.9	43.4	40.1	6.1	5.9	6.0
Ph.D. or equivalent	54.5	53.9	44.2	5.5	5.8	6.2	42.3	47.1	44.8	5.5	5.6	5.4
M.D. and Ph.D. or equivalent	44.7	42.0	50.0	5.4	5.5	6.2	44.6	49.7	46.5	5.5	5.6	6.4
Men	44.0	42.6	35.6	5.1	5.7	6.2	42.9	44.2	39.8	5.7	5.9	6.1
Women	36.0	32.1	26.4	5.7	6.2	6.5	31.0	32.6	34.1	6.0	6.2	6.4
White (not Hispanic/Latino)	46.3	42.6	34.9	5.2	5.8	6.2	42.7	43.9	40.2	5.7	5.9	6.1
Non-white	32.6	30.9	25.2	5.4	5.8	6.3	35.0	36.0	31.1	5.9	6.0	6.2
Tenure track	71.8	51.6	46.8	5.0	5.7	6.2	52.2	51.2	48.6	5.6	5.9	6.0
Non-tenure track	46.4	33.8	28.0	5.4	5.9	6.3	34.5	32.3	29.2	5.5	5.9	6.3

Words to the Wise

- Demystify the promotion process by reading the faculty handbook, studying websites, reviewing template letters to referees, and clinical/teaching evaluation forms. Understand policies regarding promotion clock extensions and early promotions.
- Collect and organize contributions cumulatively through an e-portfolio.
- Gather perspectives from mentors and colleagues but identify one person—usually the department chair (or designate)—who will serve as the authoritative interpreter of criteria and of the promotion review process.
- Attend and actively participate in career development and promotion workshops.
- Meet annually with department chair to track progress toward promotion. Incorporate feedback from midterm review into action plan and refine the timeline that leads to a robust body of scholarship, teaching, and clinical contributions by the time the promotion package is submitted.
- Understand the timing of the promotion review and when candidate materials are due.
- Circulate promotion package to mentors and colleagues for review and advice.
- Determine which, if any, information can be provided post-promotion package submission (e.g., accepted publications, awards, grants).

Ask Your Mentor or Colleagues

- What should you do when the guidance you are receiving from your mentor conflicts with your own sense of what is needed for promotion?
- What was the most important feedback you received from your midterm review?

(continued)

(continued)

- How did you find the right voice in writing your candidate's statement for two audiences: experts in your field and faculty from other disciplines?
- What is the most valuable lesson you learned from the promotion process?

Appendix: Sample Promotion Process Timeline

Clock	Tasks
14 Months before promotion	Dean's office and department confer about the promotion review
13 Months before promotion	Dean's office sends email notifying the faculty member that the review has commenced, copying the department chair. Faculty member provides CV, candidate's statement, list of current and former trainees, suggested referees, teaching evaluations, and sample publications
12 Months before promotion	Department identifies the review committee members. Department reviews candidate's materials and requests revisions, if necessary
11 Months before promotion	Department compiles referee list and, if appropriate, the comparison peer list. Department solicits evaluations from internal and external referees and trainees. Department chair makes writing assignments for all sections of the promotion file requiring written text (scholarship, clinical duties, teaching duties, etc.)
10 Months before promotion	Department awaits receipt of referee and trainee letters and sends reminders, if necessary
9 Months before promotion	Department receives most or all of the referee and trainee letters. Sections on scholarship, clinical and teaching activities are finalized
8 Months before promotion	Department receives all referee and trainee letters. All written portions of the file are completed. The review committee has met or a meeting is scheduled. Post-review, the review committee provides a written evaluation of the candidate

Clock	Tasks
7 Months before promotion	Department concludes its review by any and all voting bodies. Department completes promotion file. Dean's Office reviews file and suggests revisions, if necessary
6 Months before promotion	Final version of the departmental file is prepared for review by higher levels
5 Months before promotion	School conducts review. This step may involve multiple levels of review (e.g., Appointments and Promotions Committee, Dean)
1–4 Months before promotion	University conducts review. (This step may involve multiple levels of review, e.g., university-wide review committee, Provost, President). Candidate is informed of the promotion decision
Promotion becomes effective	Formal notification letters are issued. Administrative systems are updated

References

1. Trower CA, Gallagher AS. Perspectives on what pre-tenure faculty want and what six research universities provide. Cambridge, MA: Harvard Graduate School of Education; 2008.
2. JAMA Instructions for Authors. http://jama.ama-assn.org/site/misc/ifora. xhtml#AuthorshipCriteriaandContributionsandAuthorshipForm.

How to Develop an Educator's Portfolio

19

Deborah Simpson

Educators seeking academic promotion must provide documentation that they have achieved the academic standards and expectations for faculty as scholars.

Documentation approaches for medical educators have evolved from the concepts and principles that emerged from the Carnegie Foundation for the Advancement of Teaching, beginning with Scholarship Reconsidered [1] and Scholarship Assessed [2]. These scholars first legitimized teaching as one of four functions of the professoriate. Then, using existing standards and criteria recommended by journals, funding agencies and academic promotion guidelines, Glassick and his colleagues [2] outlined the domains associated with a scholarly approach. As teachers, these domains mirror approaches that have evolved from the field of education and include clear goals, adequate preparation, appropriate methods, significant results, effective presentation, and reflective critique. Over time institutions have adopted these domains and defined associated standards for documentation and evaluation of excellence in teaching [3]. This chapter will use these six domain areas as a framework for stepwise development and presentation of an Educator's Portfolio.

D. Simpson, Ph.D. (✉)
Academic Administration, Aurora Health Care,
1020 N. 12th St. Suite 5120, Milwaukee, WI, USA
e-mail: deb.simpson@aurora.org

© Springer International Publishing Switzerland 2016
L.W. Roberts (ed.), *The Clinician Educator Guidebook*,
DOI 10.1007/978-3-319-27980-0_19

Clear Goals

An Educator's Portfolio (EP) for academic promotion has one clear and specific goal which is to present the *best* evidence of excellence as an educator–scholar. While meeting the education mission requires all faculty, an individual faculty member's ability to achieve excellence in teaching, curriculum development, learner assessment, advising/mentoring, and educational leadership [4] is often challenged by other roles, responsibilities, and expertise. Typically, promotion-oriented EPs include two to three educator activity categories and are dependent on the faculty member's role and institution-specific academic promotion guidelines.

Presenting the best evidence of one's role as an educator–scholar can be accomplished using a three-step process:

Step #1. The first objective in creating an EP is to identify educator activity categories in which you spend your time. The easiest approach is to use the worksheet provided in Appendix 1 of this chapter. Spend 5–10 min writing the keywords for each of the activities in which you regularly engage as a teacher/educator in worksheet column #1. As you write, check your calendar to ensure that you include things like admission committee meetings, graduate studies council, rating a resident's performance, or meeting with a trainee to discuss career plans.

Step #2. Next, connect each activity to the five commonly accepted educator activity categories by placing a checkmark in the column that it best matches: Teach = Teaching (e.g., presented grand rounds, attending onwards, small group facilitator, lab instructor); Curr Dev = Curriculum Development (e.g., a unit of instruction on patient safety, a workshop on professionalism, an interactive e-learning module on scientific principles underlying geriatrics); A/M = Advising/Mentor (e.g., guiding selection of fourth year electives, reviewing resident's CV for job application, reviewing graduate student's grant application); Assess = Assessment of Learners (e.g., authoring multiple choice questions or an standardized patient checklist); Leader = Leadership and Management (e.g., course/clerkship/program director, committee charge); and Oth = Other.

Step #3. Identify your major "valued added" activity categories. Most educators spend time in roles aligned with other institutional missions including clinical care, research, and/or community engagement. Therefore most EPs demonstrate the continuous record typically needed for promotion in two to three activity categories. Review your entries to ascertain which activity categories demonstrate your major contribution(s) as an educator and then consider which of those entries are most highly valued by you and your organization. Typically portfolios have page limits (e.g., 6–10 pages). Selecting your best categories as focal points allows you to present evidence of your excellence as an educator–scholar consistent with having a clear goal/focus as an educator.

Adequate Preparation: Before Starting

Each college/university has specific guidelines for academic promotion. As mentioned in previous chapters, prior to beginning the actual development of an Educator's Portfolio, the academic physician must obtain and follow his or her institution's specific guidelines, procedures, and timelines. While your chair or a senior faculty member should provide guidance about the formal and tacit processes associated with promotion documentation, it is still incumbent on each faculty member to fully understand the guidelines and prepare promotion materials consistent with those standards. If the institution does not have specific guidelines related to documenting contributions as an educator, check with the faculty affairs office and faculty who have been successfully promoted and ask for their guidance regarding appropriate documentation.

Obtain examples of successful educator portfolios from colleagues locally and nationally. Often institutions post-examples on their internal websites in the same location as the promotion guidelines [5]. Other resources with examples are also available through professional societies and medical education organizations [6].

Adequate preparation allows faculty to demonstrate that they have met the standards of an education scholar. All faculty are expected to demonstrate their abilities as scholars, defined as advancement of their field through teaching, discovery, integration, and application, by drawing from the established body of knowledge in the area of interest [1]. Therefore, the EP must demonstrate how teaching practices, curriculum, assessment tools, and advising/mentoring approaches have been informed by what is already known in medical education. For example, when you teach, do you select the teaching methods (e.g., participant response system, mobile app, virtual patient, PowerPoint presentation) and then prepare your instruction informed by the best practices in the field? This is important because as a faculty member seeking promotion, it is expected that the portfolio will provide evidence demonstrating that the faculty member has met the adequate preparation criteria as an educator–scholar.

The number of books, journals, and peer-reviewed forums in medical/health professions education is expanding and is easily accessible to faculty, ensuring that your approach to education is evidence-based [7]. Typically, educators read selected medical education journals sponsored by national and international associations including Academic Medicine (Association of American Medical Colleges—AAMC), Medical Science Educator (International Association of Medical Science Educators—IAMSE), Medical Education (Association for the Study of Medical Education—ASME), and Medical Teacher (Association of Medical Education in Europe—AMEE). In addition, educators often read journals keyed to trainee level (e.g., Journal of Graduate Medical Education, Journal of Continuing Education in the Health Professions) and specialty/discipline-specific journals addressing education which are now available in almost every health profession medical specialty. Often your library has purchased subscriptions to these journals and current issues are available on the web to browse.

Consistent with the Carnegie Foundation for the Advancement of Teaching's expanded view of scholarship, educators have available to them other forms of shared knowledge ranging from curriculum materials and learner assessment instruments to faculty development workshops and advising guides. As with journals, some repositories house peer-reviewed materials across the continuum of medical education, such as MedEDPORTAL, while others are specialty/topic-specific repositories such as POGOe for geriatrics and PERC for Prevention Education. These repositories are easily accessed through the web using any search engine. Some may require log-in but most are available at no charge.

In summary, the adequate preparation standard requires that for each educator activity category, the academic physician is able to document how his or her work was informed by and builds on what is already known in medical education.

Appropriate Methods

An Educator's Portfolio is considered an *asynchronous instructional material*, enabling faculty to communicate their achievements with others at a time and place that is convenient for them. For instance, academic promotion reviewers usually independently review each promotion packet and then meet as a member of a committee (e.g., A&P committee) in a closed session to discuss the portfolio and make a determination as to the faculty member's readiness for promotion. Therefore, the EP must be designed to effectively "teach" reviewers (e.g., promotion committee, department chairs, future employers) about the roles and impact one has as a teacher, curriculum developer, assessor of learner performance, adviser/mentor, and educational leader.

Building on one's adequate preparation, the method(s) one selects to teach his or her EP audience (e.g., promotion committee members) should be informed by the successful EPs used by colleagues at the institution with whom one shares common activity categories (e.g., advising/mentoring). Review institution-specific promotion guidelines to ascertain how the activity descriptions within each category are to be listed within the curriculum vitae. Then, use the EP to provide evidence documenting excellence to support and compliment the CV entries.

Typically, the description of an activity within a category begins with the date, educator role, topic, learner audience, and frequency. These activity descriptions are often organized within each activity category by using sub-headers associated with trainee level (e.g., medical student, resident, continuing professional education), trainee specialty/program (e.g., Medicine-Geriatric Fellowship), and school/college (e.g., Graduate School of Biomedical Sciences, College of Nursing, School of Medicine). The use of sub-headers within an activity category helps the reader understand the array of audiences and the topics taught, which emphasizes the breadth and depth of initiatives in each activity category. For example, a CV entry under the "Teaching" activity category in a CV or EP might contain two or three sub-headers: Medical Students, Residents, and Continuing Professional Education. The activity is then succinctly described. If the faculty member repeatedly teaches the same topic in a clerkship or residency program, the entry then has the inclusive dates, the faculty role (e.g., instructor, facilitator, preceptor, attending, lab, presenter), the program (e.g., clerkship, course, CME offering, graduate school), the topic(s), how many learners and frequency as shown below under two teaching activity sub-header audiences:

Teaching—medical students	
10.2009–present	Presenter: M3 family medicine core clerkship, functional assessment in older adult patients
	1 h/month/12 month/year; 30–35 students/month
Teaching—residents	
10.2011–present	Simulation lab instructor: integrated surgery block curriculum for PGY1s, post-op paracentesis in geriatric patient
	2 h/year; 16 residents from general surgery, plastics, urology and surgery PA students

If institution-specific standards provide limited guidance or are flexible, an alternative is to provide the description of the each category activity along with the evidence using the accepted scholarship standards as the organizing framework (see Appendix 2 for illustrative examples in learner assessment, mentoring/advising, and educational leadership for Drs. Anatoly and Vladimir).

After one has competed an initial draft of the entries associated with each of one's valued educator activity categories, it is helpful to have a colleague familiar with one's work review the portfolio draft. Often the colleague will identify missing activities such as LCME Workgroup on Medical Student Education (Educational Leadership) and/or guiding a resident through his or her scholarly project requirement (Advising/Mentoring). Documenting all of one's activities is important to demonstrate excellence as an educator.

Significant Results

An Educator's Portfolio provides an opportunity to provide evidence of one's effectiveness as an educator–scholar. This may include presentation of data such as teacher effectiveness ratings compared to one's peer cohort, trainee evaluations of a new curriculum unit, trainee examination performance benchmarked to the national mean where possible, accreditation site visitor commentary and judgments regarding the overall quality of a program, leadership accomplishments, and reliability and validity of an assessment instrument you developed. The list will extend as the faculty member thinks about the products and impact of his or her work as an educator.

Where does the academic physician find the evidence to demonstrate his or her excellence as an educator–scholar? Colleges and universities often have an education resource office that manages evaluation data, providing comparative data about courses, clerkships, rotations, advising, and teaching effectiveness. As accreditation organizations often require documentation that faculty teaching is evaluated, these data may be collected using the same online management systems used by faculty to submit grades. Often evaluation results are provided to faculty, course/program directors, and other stakeholders on an annual basis along with a comparison to an appropriate cohort (e.g., other teachers in the program/department). If one has misplaced this data, it may be retrievable by checking with the originating office or program. It is important to maintain this information over time in an e-file or file box that one can readily access as one is preparing for promotion. Trying to locate this information at the last minute introduces avoidable stress that can complicate one's efforts to present one's best work.

It is imperative that the educator–scholar obtain through institutional resources or through his or her own initiatives, data about the effectiveness of his or her activities. Sometimes this requires the faculty member to advocate within a department or program that the information be centrally collected so that it is not biased and can be benchmarked. If that is not possible, it is the faculty member's responsibility as an educator–scholar to systematically design an appropriate data collection and tracking approach. The first place to start in designing one's own approach is to review the literature and search the educational repositories for established tools and methods.

Effective Presentation

Attention to organization, accuracy, clarity (including the absence of grammatical and spelling errors), along with the appropriate utilization of visual displays are hallmarks of a strong portfolio. Be sure to select the most effective presentation methods (graphs, figures, flow diagrams, bulleted narratives) for the type of information you are presenting and appropriate to the targeted reviewers (e.g., level of knowledge about education, time available). Build on your strengths in selecting and preparing written materials that you use in face-to-face and online education.

Once you have completed your portfolio, ask several colleagues to review. Often it is best if you meet and ask them to "think out loud" as they read, so that you can determine if they are interpreting your narratives and visual displays as you intended. They may offer additional activity entries to strengthen one of your categories and suggest a data set that you had not considered. Be direct; ask your colleagues to provide constructive feedback to enhance the likelihood that your portfolio will achieve its goal, which is to effectively present best evidence of your excellence as an educator–scholar.

Reflective Critique

John Cotton Dana, the influential American librarian, once wrote "He who dares to teach must never cease to learn." From Donald Shön's now classic, Educating the Reflective Practitioner [8] to Lee Shulman's Signature Pedagogies in the Professions [9], the role of reflection as one of the common cross-cutting forms of instruction is emphasized. Stephen Brookfield argues that the distinguishing feature of critical reflection for teachers is its focus on "hunting assumptions" about what worked in our educational programs, what students did or did not learn, and how we can improve [10]. Without testing and exploring assumptions about teaching and learning, teachers and learners are at risk as they may cease to learn.

The inclusion of critical reflection as a final standard for judging educator–scholars provides an opportunity to step back and test our assumptions about learner motivations, instructional strategies and advising approaches, educational leadership, and testing and evaluation. Recording what was learned, new questions and ideas that were sparked by preparing and reviewing the portfolio is an opportunity to contribute to what is known in our field. A faculty member's reflective critiques and testing of assumptions with new and refined goals provide a continuous record of the educator–scholar's approach that is consistent with expectations for academic promotion.

Key Concepts
- Educator's portfolio: A document that presents evidence of excellence as an educator typically organized into five activity categories: teaching, curriculum development, learner assessment, advising/mentoring, and educational leadership.
- Evidence: Data, information, facts that demonstrate your excellence including judgments by peers who have reviewed your work as an educator.
- Scholarly approach: As defined in the work emerging from the Carnegie Foundation [2], there are six elements that faculty must demonstrate as scholars in their work: clear goals, adequate preparation, appropriate methods, significant results, effective presentation, and reflective critique. The work of an educator is judged by whether it has achieved the standards of excellence associated with each element.

Celebrate Accomplishments

Every educator with whom I have worked to create a portfolio is asked the same question, "How do you feel about yourself and your contributions as an educator?" Inevitability the answer is "Yes, I am amazing and very proud of my accomplishments as an educator … and I have so many new ideas about how to improve …" Ultimately what is presented in your Educator's Portfolio should highlight your value as a teacher and reaffirm your commitment that when you teach others—including teaching promotion committee members about what you do as an educators—you also continue to learn.

Words to the Wise
- *Clear goals.* Your Educator's Portfolio has one clear and specific aim: to demonstrate that you are an outstanding educator. Its purpose is to present best evidence of your excellence as an educator–scholar to inform academic promotion/tenure decisions.
- *Adequate preparation.* Approach the preparation of your Educator's Portfolio as you would any other instructional material by first determining your objectives and then select how to present the achievement of those objectives.
- *Appropriate methods.* An Educator's Portfolio is an *asynchronous instructional material* and must be designed to effectively teach your reviewers (e.g., promotion committee, department chairs, future employer) about the roles and impact you have as a teacher, curriculum developer, assessor of learner performance, adviser/mentor, and educational leader.
- *Significant results.* Do *not* throw evidence away. Often we receive thank you notes from advisees, teaching evaluations, accreditation notification that highlights a specific activity for which you had responsibility, and an invitation to talk with colleagues about an educational

(continued)

(continued)

approach you designed. This information, when effectively presented in a portfolio, demonstrates that peers have judged your work as an educator to meet standards of excellence as an educator–scholar.

- *Effective presentation*. Give your Educator's Portfolio multiple *test runs* before you submit the final version. Circulate the portfolio draft to experienced colleagues for review and critical comment. Revise and recirculate to obtain additional feedback to ensure that it will achieve your goal.
- *Reflective critique*. Celebrate portfolio submission by taking 20 min to write a reflective critique on your strengths and opportunities for growth as an educator.

Ask Your Mentor or Colleagues
- What are the activities you do as an educator that you value and make a difference to our learners and educational mission?
- What has informed your work in education (e.g., personal experience, colleagues, literature in the field)?
- What information/evidence would demonstrate your work is high quality? Is this evidence currently available or could you obtain it in timely fashion?
- Have you shared your work with others (e.g., presented at a medical school meeting, presented at a regional conference, published in a peer review forum)?
- Have you started your Educator's Portfolio? Note, you should start the portfolio at the same time you begin to engage in any of the five educator activity categories as the time it takes to create a portfolio equals that associated with writing a manuscript for journal submission. So, get started as early as possible!

Acknowledgements

1. U.S. Department of Health and Human Services—Faculty Development in Primary Care [Grant # D55HP23197] and Wisconsin Geriatric Education Center [Grant # 6UB4HP19062].
2. Donald W. Reynolds Foundation—Next Steps in Physicians' Training in Geriatrics.
3. National Center for Research Resources & The National Center for Advancing Translational Sciences—Clinical & Translational Science Award (CTSA) program [Grant # UL1RR031973].

References

1. Boyer EL. Scholarship reconsidered: priorities of the professoriate. San Francisco, CA: Jossey-Bass Publishers; 1990.
2. Glassick CE, Huber MT, Maeroff GI. Scholarship assessed: evaluation of the professoriate. San Francisco, CA: Jossey-Bass; 1997.
3. Hutching P, Huber MT, Ciccone A. The scholarship of teaching and learning reconsidered: institutional integration and impact. San Francisco: Jossey-Bass; 2011.
4. Simpson D, Fincher RM, Hafler JP, Irby DM, Richards BF, Rosenfeld GC, Viggiano TR. Advancing educators and education by defining the components and evidence associated with educational scholarship. Med Educ. 2007;41:10002–9.
5. Faculty Development: Developing Your Educator's Portfolio at the Medical College of Wisconsin. http://www.mcw.edu/facultyaffairs/RankandTenure1/EducatorsPortfolio.htm. Accessed 19 Nov 2012.
6. AAMC Publications: Advancing Educators and Education: Defining the Components and Evidence of Educational Scholarship. https://members.aamc.org/eweb/DynamicPage.aspx?Action=Add%26ObjectKeyFrom=1A83491A-9853-4C87-86A4-F7D95601C2E2%26WebCode=PubDetailAdd%26DoNotSave=yes%26ParentObject=CentralizedOrderEntry%26ParentDataObject=Invoice%20Detail%26ivd_formkey=69202792-63d7-4ba2-bf4e-a0da41270555%26ivd_prc_prd_key=5F2DA545-DAE0-4A44-94F4-A67C316E8FED. Accessed 19 Nov 2012.
7. Annotated Bibliography of Journals for Educational Scholarship. AAMC-Regional Groups on Education Affairs-Research in Medical Education (RIME) Section. https://www.aamc.org/download/184694/data/annotated_bibliography_of_journals.pdf. Accessed 19 Nov 2012.
8. Schön D. Educating the reflective practitioner. San Francisco: Jossey-Bass; 1987.
9. Shulman LS. Signature pedagogies in the professions. Daedalus. 2005;124(3):52–9.
10. Brookfield S. Becoming a critically reflective teacher. San Francisco: Jossey-Bass; 1995.

Appendix 1: Educator's Portfolio Worksheet—3 Steps

Step #1	Step #2						Step #3	
Teacher/ educator activities list ↓	Teach	Curr dev	A/M	Assess	Leader	Oth	You value	School values

Appendix 2: Illustrative Educator Portfolio Category Examples

Section 1: Learner Assessment, Nathan Anatoly, Ph.D., Assistant Professor Physiology

Role: Director Medical Education Council on Reintegration of Sciences Underlying Medicine into Clinical Clerkships—2011–present.

Initiative: Develop an examination to provide pre–post data regarding degree to which medical students' link basic science concepts to clinical conditions

Problem	7.2011	Curriculum integration often emphasizes incorporation of clinical applications within basic science courses
		Students and faculty report little/no reintegration of sciences into required clinical rotation and gaps in geriatric focused training
Goal	9.2011	To develop a brief (<30 min) multiple choice examination to assess third year medical student's application of the basic science concepts underlying geriatric clinical conditions

(continued)

(continued)

Adequate preparation	10.2011	Literature and educational repository review identified college level geriatric-associated assessment, but no clinical to basic science-related knowledge assessment tools
		Broad based review of geriatrics resources (e.g., textbooks on geriatrics, biology of aging) → 5 basic science geriatrics concepts
		A multi-disciplinary workgroup including geriatricians reviewed the themes and confirmed their utility. Themes included: impaired homeostasis, connective tissue changes, post-mitotic tissue predilection for age changes, and immunosenescence
Methods	11.2011	Workgroup developed test blueprint: 5 "cross-cutting" geriatric-related basic science themes × 13 common geriatric conditions
		Examination consisted of 26 multiple choice questions (MCQs) as 13-item pairs: the first question assessed the clinical condition/disease/illness and the second question in the pair assessed the associated underlying basic science
Results	12.2011	50 Trainees completed examination <25 min on average
		Pre-test mean performance was 57.7 % correct (range 34–77 %)
		Overall exam reliability is in moderate range (≥0.71)
Present	3.2012	Presented to curriculum committee who approved with commendation
		Peer-reviewed abstracts presented at AAMC-central group on educational affairs and american geriatrics society
		Examination accepted in POGOe
Reflect critique	5.2012	A paired clinical and underlying science MCQ type examination provides a reliable assessment of trainees' ability to apply underlying basic science concepts to clinical geriatrics

Section 2: Mentor/Advising, Nathan Anatoly, Ph.D., Assistant Professor Physiology

Role: Advisor to medical students enrolled in physician scientist pathway, graduate students, and residents/fellows interested in aging-related clinical translational research studies.

Initiative(s): Medical school, graduate school, and education core—NIH Clinical & Translational Science Award (CTSA)

Goal	9.2009 to present	To advance advisees' ability to systematically identify, conduct, analyze, and present research findings for age-related studies
		To have advisees' accurately identify the translational research level for their study question(s) and then articulate how each question and its findings will inform work at a subsequent translation stage
Adequate prep	9.2009 to present	Continuously reviewed literature and websites associated with effective research mentoring and translational research; established RSS feed through library to receive updated citations
		Attend local CTSA sponsored training sessions on advising/mentoring
Methods	1.2010 to present	Schedule 1-on-1 meetings with interested trainees to ascertain if appropriate to begin working together
		Complete an individual learning plan with timelines, roles, and tasks for advisee and advisor
		Follow-up with advisees at regular intervals (e.g., e-mail, Google docs, FaceTime™) to evaluate progress and outline next steps
		Review document drafts
		Post-accepted abstracts and links to provide resources for translational research (in consultation with CTSA)
		Sponsor and invite all advisees and faculty colleagues to attend the monthly *Grr5* (Geriatric Research & Refreshments at 5:00 pm) to facilitate establishment of colleague network in geriatric research

(continued)

(continued)

Results	6.2011 to present	Relationships established: 15 active advisees—3 Ph.D.s, 3 MSs, 4 residents; 5 pathway students ranging from M1–3 years
		Collaboration: 4/5 pathway students working with grad students
		Graduates to date: N = 5–2 Ph.D.s (now post-docs); 1 resident (in fellowship); 2 pathway students
		Scholarship: 8 Advisee publications including 2 in translational science journals; 4 regional/national presentations; student presentation 1/5 outstanding research awards at annual American Geriatric Society annual meeting
Present	1.2012	*Grr5* presented to NIH-CTSA external advisory board as example of fostering collaborations; cited as institutional strength in follow-up report
Reflect critique	2.2012	Engaging with trainees interested in translational geriatric research is vital to advancing science and health
		Sustaining my own vitality and funding as a researcher is challenging when advisee/advisor relationships are <3 years

Section 3: Educational Leadership Isaac Vladimir, M.D., Associate Professor Emergency Medicine

Role: Chair medical student curriculum committee (2010–2012).

Initiative: Incentive environment and accountability in medical student education

Problem	8.2010	Educational resources not optimally aligned with faculty effort needed to achieve educational goals
		Expectations for clerkship directors and protected time varied by department
		Enterprise activity performance systems (EAPS) do not include teaching or educational leadership metrics

(continued)

Goal	9.2010	Establish and incorporate systems to recognize and reward teaching within financial model
		Establish job expectations including protected time for directors of required clerkships
Adequate preparation	10.2010	Review local data from clerkship leaders and LCME requirements for teaching and time expectations
		Reviewed policies from other medical schools, national clerkship director standards, and literature on financial structures to support medical student education
Effective methods	11.2010	Retreat held with campus education leaders to discuss problem and collate recommendations
		Developed draft document on mandatory clerkship expectations and protected time
		Worked toward consensus document with the curriculum committee, faculty governance, clinical chairs, and the dean
Results and presentation	3.2011	Presented findings to dean who expressed support for aligning revenue with teaching effort
		Clinical chairs and dean unanimously approved the clerkship director job expectation document which included department support for protected time
	10.2011	Dean and faculty council approve utilizing MCW financial support towards departments as revenue support for departmental clerkship curricular management/leadership
	1.2012	List of teaching metrics provided to the chief financial officer for the enterprise activity performance system
Reflect critique	2.2012	Consistent cross department expectations for clerkship directors and metrics within EAPS resource allocation
		Sustaining momentum will be challenging with transitions in leadership and competing resources demands

How to Build a National Reputation for Academic Promotion

20

Sidney Zisook and Laura B. Dunn

At most academic institutions, promotion from assistant to associate level in clinical, research, or any other academic track requires the individual to demonstrate that one has developed an outstanding local and regional reputation in an area of expertise. Promotion to professor requires developing an excellent national, if not international, reputation. As there is no single best route to achieving a strong academic reputation, this chapter focuses on principles that help early career academicians to best position themselves to seize and capitalize on opportunities to attain this goal. Obstacles that can impede achievement of a national reputation also are discussed.

Start Early, If You Can

If you don't know where you are going, you might wind up someplace else.

Yogi Berra

When selecting a residency or fellowship, consider not only short-term needs to get excellent clinical training in a program

2020

L.B. Dunn, M.D. (✉)
Department of Psychiatry, University of California, San Francisco,
401 Parnassus Ave., San Francisco, CA, USA
e-mail: laura.dunn@ucsf.edu

© Springer International Publishing Switzerland 2016
L.W. Roberts (ed.), *The Clinician Educator Guidebook*,
DOI 10.1007/978-3-319-27980-0_20

where residents appear satisfied and respected, but also longer term goals of preparing for an academic career. A resident who aspires to a successful academic career that will, by necessity, require the development of an excellent national reputation would be wise to select a program with faculty members who have attained strong national reputations. Some programs are more successful as launching pads for competitive fellowships or academic appointments. The best way to find out is to ask focused questions of training directors, residents, fellows, and junior faculty at the interviews such as "Do trainees have opportunities, dedicated time, mentorship, and available resources to develop areas of interest most important to them?" "What do residents do after graduation?" "How many go into the most competitive fellowships?" "Where do they go for fellowships?" "How many graduates assume leadership positions in the field and develop national or international reputations?"

For trainees interested in basic, translational, or clinical research, a research-oriented department with top scientists on the faculty bears careful consideration. For the trainee aspiring to develop a reputation as an academic clinician-educator, a program with a clinical scholar or clinical educator track may be especially appealing. For someone who is undecided about post-training plans, a program with a broad range of opportunities and mentors is ideal.

At the faculty level, it may be more difficult to select the ideal program as faculty positions may be more limited. Since the best predictor of the future is the past, it may be wise to visit a program more than once to learn how successful early-career faculty have been in developing their reputations and attaining advancement. Some questions to consider are "Do junior faculty feel satisfied and valued?" "Do they foresee opportunities for advancement?" "Are adequate resources available—including mentorship, time and encouragement to build their academic portfolios and reputations?"

Do your homework to evaluate whether junior faculty have advanced to senior leadership and academic positions, either at the same institution or elsewhere. It is also important to evaluate the degree to which faculty have developed or are developing regional, national, and international reputations. Some questions to consider are "Do junior faculty participate actively in national and international organizations?" "Do they attend meetings of these organizations?" "Do they feel that they have colleagues who are looking out for them?" "Do they have mentors who introduce them to others in the field or otherwise help them to become known?"

Other departmental and institutional factors can affect your ability to develop a national reputation, but such factors may take more investigation. These include the overall functioning and stability of the department and the role of the Chair and other senior leadership. A department without a permanent chair, or one in severe financial difficulty, may not be as conducive for the development of academic faculty. Some Chairs see the development of early-career faculty—introducing them to key players in their field of interest, facilitating invitations to appropriate national organizations, helping with grant applications, protecting them from too much service—as a core feature of their main mission, while others are less focused on or dedicated to faculty development. Therefore, it may be important to know how generative and dedicated to faculty development the Chair and other departmental leaders are when choosing between job offers.

There are several "tracks" available for academic physicians. Navigating each pathway requires knowledge of what is available, the local institutional "culture," and the process and criteria most relevant to the chosen path [1]. The hierarchy of faculty ranks in many academic medical centers include moving up the ladder from Instructor to Assistant Professor to Associate Professor and finally to Professor. In many centers, the qualifiers, "clinical" or "research," or their equivalents, may be attached to the title, for example, Clinical Assistant Professor or Research Professor. Table 20.1 describes a general overview of what promotion committees look for in each major academic "track." For the research scholar, for example, the rank of Research Professor (sometimes just called Professor) is the goal, and promotion is based on a strong national and international reputation in research. To a lesser extent, teaching and possibly even clinical skills may be important. The focus is more on publishing manuscripts and obtaining peer-reviewed funding than it is on seeing patients.

Table 20.1 Academic tracks

		Track		
		Research scholar	Clinical scholar/ educator	Clinical
Accomplish- ments/reputation	Example title	Research professor or professor of X	Professor of clinical X	Clinical professor
Research (manuscripts/ grants)		☑☑☑☑	☑☑	☑
Education/ training		☑☑	☑☑☑☑	☑☑
Clinical		☑☑	☑☑	☑☑☑☑

☑☑☑☑ = strong reputation required for promotion
☑☑ = some accomplishments may be required or desired
☑☑ = not usually required

The educator and clinical scholar generally are required to build a strong reputation as a teacher and clinician, and less so as an independent investigator. As mentioned in Chap. 17, teaching innovations and creative curricular development may be more important than original research or the number of publications in this track. Finally, the clinician is judged primarily on clinical excellence, often less so on teaching and minimally on research. The sooner you know the idiosyncrasies of each track at your institution, the more likely you are to take the appropriate steps to ensure success in achieving excellent reputations in the field, leading to timely promotions and the satisfaction, prestige and awards that go with them.

Follow Your Passion, Once You Find It

Don't ask what the world needs. Rather ask—what makes you come alive? Then go and do it! Because what the world needs is people who have come alive.

Howard Thurman

Being a physician remains a privileged and honored profession. Few professions offer as many choices—to be a healer, a teacher, a scientist, an expert in medical law, a bioinformatics specialist, to name a few—for a fulfilling and purposeful career. However, it can be challenging to find which among these many possibilities best matches your interests, talents, and temperament. For those who choose careers in academic medicine, the menu can be overwhelming.

While it is important to focus on the areas of academic medicine (e.g., clinical work, teach, research, and community service), it is helpful to understand that whatever early decisions are made, they are not written in stone—people do change directions and adjust their relative emphases on roles over time. It is not unusual for an M.D./Ph.D. to enter a residency fully intent on setting the basic science research world on fire when they graduate, only to find they love caring for patients and to shift to a more clinically oriented career. Similarly, it is not unusual for someone with minimal or no background in research to become excited by the world of discovery during their training and ultimately develop into an outstanding investigator. Thus, early career academicians are faced with the task of discovering their unique academic passions, following them, while being open and flexible to emerging attractions.

Strive for Everyday Excellence

The best preparation for tomorrow is to do today's work superbly well.

William Osler

If there is one *sine qua non* for building a national reputation, it is establishing a local reputation as a reliable colleague and a trustworthy team player who always strives towards excellence. The ACGME competencies provide a useful framework: (1) knowledge (in your general discipline and specific field of concentration), (2) clinical skills (for purposes of professional careers in academic medicine, this can be broadened to include also teaching skills and research skills), (3) practice-based learning and improvement (be at the cutting edge and do what is necessary to stay there),

(4) interpersonal and communication skills (in day-to-day work with colleagues, students, and the public as well as in disseminating work verbally and in writing), (5) professionalism (a commitment to adhering to ethical principles, respect for others, and personal integrity), and (6) systems-based practice (working within the unique intricacies of available resources and the "culture" of your department, university, and national organizations). Attention to each of these areas is much more fruitful than focusing on the more expansive goal of attaining a "national reputation" and is an effective strategy towards academic success.

A dream doesn't become reality through magic; it takes sweat, determination and hard work.

(Colin Powell)

Being an academic physician is hard work. Few academicians begin their careers as fully funded investigators, and no one starts a career as a fully funded teacher or clinician. Thus, academic faculty frequently have several institutional responsibilities and often find themselves with multiple roles including front-line clinical treatment and care. Moreover, faculty often have responsibilities related to patients, students, colleagues, supervisors, mentors, organizations, and communities and to their families. They may be surprised to find themselves working even harder as junior faculty than they did as residents. If they want to make their mark as investigators, they may have to write manuscripts and grant applications in the evenings and on weekends. It may be wise to have frank discussions with your life partner about such demands to make sure that each of you is prepared for the sacrifices. Despite the hard work, when the chair requests a patient to be seen, or your mentor asks for a review of a manuscript he or she has just written, as junior faculty the answer should almost always be, "Happily," or "Of course." For the most part, bargaining and negotiating are skills to use as one moves into mid-career and later.

Say Yes

I only have "yes" men around me. Who needs "no" men?

Mae West

While it is always an asset to be collegial and a good team player, it is especially important early in your career to take advantage of every possible opportunity. The first step in developing a national reputation is developing a local one, and the trainee or early-career faculty member who is viewed as eagerly doing more than his or her share is well on the way. A resident who wants to be nominated for one of the many scholarships, fellowship, travel awards, and other honors available to residents generally does so by being considered a "good citizen" of the residency and department. Personal qualities are every bit as important, sometimes more so, than native intelligence or even accomplishments in getting recognized and promoted. One of the key personal qualities is being considered a giving team player. For both house staff and faculty, the individual who looks at a request more as an opportunity than a burden has an advantage. Even better is the person who does not wait to be asked, but who volunteers for service such as teaching, seeing a difficult patient, serving on committees, consulting to another service, and covering for a colleague in need. Rarely does a promotion committee's recommendation omit "teamwork." Regardless of how much time you lament that too much of your time is spent in front of your computer instead of with patients or students, or that you are too tethered to your cell phone and pager when you would prefer to be free to think, read or, importantly, relax, professionalism demands that you answer pages promptly, return calls, and respond to emails. Part of the reputation you build along the way is directly related to day-to-day communications, electronic or otherwise.

Just Say No (Thanks)

It comes from saying no to 1,000 things to make sure we don't get on the wrong track or try to do too much. We're always thinking about new markets we could enter, but it's only by saying no that you can concentrate on the things that are really important.

Steve Jobs

There comes a time when "Yes, thank you; more, please" cannot remain the default reply to all requests. No one can do it all, which often requires learning the art of saying "No, thank you." To protect your time and to focus on unique academic passions and career goals, it becomes important to recognize limits and eliminate extraneous pursuits. Books have been written on the gentle art of saying no [2]. Usually a straightforward "Thanks for the offer, but I just have too much on my plate right now" will do. There is no reason to apologize for not being a super hero; none of us are. If someone such as a Chair, the Dean or another important "boss" is asking, and especially if he is insistent, it sometimes helps to review with them other commitments and enlist their help in re-prioritizing. You may be able to reach a compromise, and an initial "No, thank you" may turn into "Can I get back to you in a few weeks? or, I'll try to get to it next month." But sometimes, it is incumbent on the individual to respect his or her own priorities and time (for more on "saying no" see Chap. 18).

Find the Right Mentor

A self-taught man usually has a poor teacher and a worse student.

Henny Youngman

The right mentor can help pave the road to an outstanding reputation in many ways. The prime responsibility of a mentor is to help guide the mentee to a rewarding and successful career in academic medicine [3]. Research has found that mentorship in academic medicine has an important influence on personal development and productivity [4], perhaps especially for women [5] and minorities [6]. Mentorship can take many forms. For the research scientist, this may entail help in developing a research focus, finding grant support, publishing, and presenting findings. Mentors can also help the up-and-coming researcher find ongoing projects to get involved in or datasets to mine while they wait for their own research to be funded or to begin yielding results.

For the educator, a mentor may focus on helping the mentee develop teaching skills and finding opportunities to teach both locally and to broader audiences. Mentors also assist mentees in getting involved in curriculum development, presenting their creative ideas in other settings outside the department and university, and navigating the institutional system to find teaching and administrative positions in the medical school or department.

For the clinical scholar, a mentor might help the mentee learn to turn a clinical conundrum into a researchable question or literature review, and a challenging patient into a publishable case report. Effective mentors are also good role models. They help their mentees learn when to say "Yes" and when to decline. They may also provide advice on difficult topics such as balancing work, family, leisure, and health. An important role mentors have is advocating for and promoting their mentees in the department, medical school, and national organizations. An effective mentor often introduces mentees to other potential mentors, supervisors, and collaborators. Often multiple mentors may provide complimentary roles. Perhaps most important, mentors provide guidance on what it takes to develop an outstanding reputation and get promoted.

Sign Up

I don't know what your destiny will be, but one thing I know: the only ones among you who will be really happy are those who have sought and found how to serve.

Albert Schweitzer

Initiating, sustaining, and nurturing connections with others, referred to as "networking," generally require active participation in local and national conferences and organizations. Be proactive. Awards, fellowships, and scholarships are available for residents, fellows, junior residents, and junior faculty. Do not assume that just because your training director, mentor, or chair has not nominated you that you are not competitive, or even that they know what is out there. Ask. If they do not know, ask other faculty members from inside and outside your department, colleagues, and acquaintances from other programs. Be creative about searching for awards and fellowships, check society websites and the NIH website. When you hear about awards or fellowships, let your immediate supervisors know of your interest.

At meetings, it is useful to seek out established investigators and "experts" and introduce yourself to let them know of your interest in their work. Junior scholars are often surprised at how accessible the academic "superstars" are, and how willing they are to offer advice and guidance. When possible, mentors can play an important role in making introductions and facilitating these connections. A second way to meet established academicians is to present a talk or poster at national conferences. Some of the most interesting and intense discussions occur during poster sessions—often more so than during more formal presentations or talks. A third way is to participate in workshops and symposia. Not only does this give the presenter a chance to disseminate her work, it also fosters connections with other investigators. Also, take the initiative to organize and submit a symposium, asking established experts to join can be a great way to be seen as a leader and to build long-lasting relationships.

Fellowships and Training Grants

Training is everything. The peach was once a bitter almond; cauliflower is nothing but cabbage with a college education.

Mark Twain

While clinical positions are often available immediately after residencies, an important intermediary step for the budding research scholars is a research fellowship. The "right" fellowship provides training in necessary research skills and mentorship regarding academic and general career development. It provides you with time to build your CV, attain research support before applying for academic appointments, and obtain opportunities to network to further develop your academic reputation. There a variety of postdoctoral research training programs available to residency training graduates [7]. Among them, NIH funded institutional T32 Training Grants (http://grants.nih.gov/training/nrsa.htm) providing stipends and an institutional allowance, are specifically designed to provide young scientists with experience in research methodology and to train the next generation of physician scholars. Often, one of the key goals in T32 or other research fellowships is for the young investigator to emerge with research funding, such as a K award. The NIH career development (K series) is a key vehicle for successful progression to independent investigator (http://grants.nih.gov/training/careerdevelopmentawards.htm). A K award validates for the candidate, professional colleagues, and the funding agency that the recipient has made a serious commitment to life as a researcher [8]. These typically provide a much higher level of salary support than other research grants and require at least a 75 % time commitment, which allows junior investigators the necessary protected time to develop their own research programs.

Write

Either write something worth reading or do something worth writing.

Benjamin Franklin

For many academic physicians, manuscripts and grants are the key currencies for promotion, for building a reputation, and for disseminating creative accomplishments. For clinical scholars and research scientists, the quality and quantity of peer-reviewed manuscripts are important components of building a reputation and at least some of the publications should be in high impact journals. In the earliest stages, contributing to manuscripts, even in a limited way in multi-authored papers, represents a good start, but eventually some first authored papers are necessary, both for promotion and for building a reputation. Sometimes, only the first author is remembered. Later in your career, being last, or "senior" author conveys even more status than first authorship, as it communicates being the "leader of the team."

Embrace Failure

I've failed over and over and over again in my life and that is why I succeed.

Michael Jordan

Success consists of going from failure to failure without loss of enthusiasm.

Winston Churchill

There is no way to succeed in academics without taking risks. When submitting a paper for publication, it is often wise to aim for a journal that is more widely read, or more academically prestigious, than where you think it is likely to get accepted. For one thing, you never know and for another you often receive feedback to improve the quality of the work. It can be the equivalent of free expert supervisory or mentor advice. Requests for revision or even frank rejections must be seen as opportunities to do better rather than personal criticisms. Most reviewers do not feel they are doing jobs if they just praise a submission or accept it outright, therefore, even the most established academicians rarely receive immediate acceptances on their initial submissions. This is even truer of grant applications, where the vast majority of submissions never get funded and those that do achieve funding often do so only after one or two revised applications. Trying may mean that you may sometimes fail but, more importantly, that you will also sometimes succeed.

Words to the Wise
- Strive for excellence, not for reputation.
- Be known as a good friend, classmate, and colleague first and foremost.
- Learn to focus on what is most important to one's academic passions and values, even if it means sometimes saying "no."
- Publish—often and well.
- Network.
- Volunteer.
- Collaborate.
- Reach out to others, including to faculty more junior than you and to the public.

Ask Your Mentor or Colleagues
- What do I need to do here to succeed?
- What is most likely to derail me from developing a national reputation? How can I best avoid those road-blocks? Are there examples of either you can share with me?
- How do I ensure time to write and for my own research (or teaching)?
- Who should I get to know here? Locally? Nationally? Internationally? Can you help me meet them? If not you, who?
- What organizations should I join?
- What awards, scholarships, and fellowships are available for me?
- How important is it for me to review manuscripts? Research proposals? If important, can you help me let people know I am available?

References

1. Buchanan GR. Academic promotion and tenure: a user's guide for junior faculty members. Am Soc Hematol. 2009;2009:736–41.
2. Grzyb JE, Chandler R. The nice factor: the art of saying no. London: Fusion; 2008.
3. Jotkowitz A, Clarfield M. Mentoring in internal medicine. Eur J Intern Med. 2006;17:399–401.
4. Sambunjak D, Straus SE, Marusić A. Mentoring in academic medicine. J Am Med Assoc. 2006;296: 1103–15.
5. McGuire LK, Bergen MR, Polan ML. Career advancement for women faculty in a U.S. school of medicine: perceived needs. Acad Med. 2004;79:319–25.
6. Benson CA, Morahan PS, Sachdeva AK, Richman RC. Effective faculty preceptoring and mentoring during reorganization of an academic medical center. Med Teach. 2002;7:717–24.
7. Podskalny JM. NIH early career funding opportunities. Gastroenterology. 2011;141:1159–962.
8. Kupfer DJ, Schatzberg AF, Grochocinski VJ, Dunn LO, Kelley KA, O'Hara RM. The Career Development Institute for Psychiatry: an innovative, longitudinal program for physician-scientists. Acad Psychiatry. 2009;33(4):313–8.

Index